Blanket of Hope

THROUGH FAITH
AND FITNESS

To Greg & Ann,
God Bless You Both

Linda C. Hillsman

Linda

A Blanket of Hope Through Faith and Fitness
by Linda Hillsman

Published by
Linda C. Hillsman
La Grange Park, IL, USA
www.lindahillsman.com

Copyright ©2014 Linda Hillsman
All rights reserved.

Author's Notes
Due to the author's discretion, and to protect the privacy of those mentioned in this book, some of the names have been changed.

Disclaimer
Please seek medical clearance from your doctor before performing any of the exercises and/or stretches included in this book. If at any time you feel discomfort or pain, please stop the exercise or stretch and call your doctor. Please discontinue the exercise or stretch if you feel a sudden change in your heart rate, abnormal blood pressure, or you feel faint. Please either call your doctor, emergency care facility, or dial 911. When performing any of the exercises or stretches listed in this book, the participant agrees to hold harmless Linda Hillsman, or any of her family members, from any and all claims, demands, damages, rights of action, or causes of action, present or future, arising out of or connected to participation in any or all stretches or exercises included in this book.

Cover art painting: Vicky Tesmer, Tres Jolie Art, Inc., www.vickytesmer.com
Cover and interior design: Cathy Davis, www.DavisCreative.com
Photography: Carolina Menapace

ISBN: 978-1502770134

TABLE OF CONTENTS

Acknowledgments

First, I'd like to thank God for all that He has given me. He was my anchor when I needed strength; He was my light when I saw nothing but darkness; He showed me love through my family and friends; and, His empowerment covered me with a blanket of hope.

To my mom, Nancy, your love for God has taught me to pray to Him with all my heart. To my father, Ernie, your love and kindness kept me nourished throughout my chemotherapy and radiation treatments.

To my husband, Rich, and children, Caitlin, Dana and Michael, your love and support meant everything to me and were never ending.

To my sister-in-law, Jean, thank you for your technical assistance and formatting ideas. You helped turn my dream into a reality.

To Carolina Menapace, thank you for your help with the photography. Your creative eye, through the lens of a camera, inspired me to move forward with this book.

Many thanks to Cathy Davis of Davis Creative, your guidance and help with the printing of this book was immeasurable.

Special thanks to Vicky Tesmer. Your artwork, which became the cover of this book, was the perfect finishing touch.

To women who have breast cancer, this book is dedicated to you.

Introduction

No one ever wants to hear the words you have breast cancer, or the tumor is malignant. Unfortunately, it happens to more women than we realize. Sometimes we feel a lump in our breast, sometimes we don't. Sometimes it sneaks up, robbing us of our feeling of security, proving that we are vulnerable. However, it doesn't have to get the best of us. In fact, a new life can actually begin at the moment of diagnosis. This book takes you through my spiritual and physical journey prior to my diagnosis of breast cancer, and through post-treatment. Each chapter contains my lesson learned that focuses on the bright side. At the end of every chapter, you will find my prayer for you asking God to bless you. The last two chapters include exercises to aid in your physical healing and questions to help you navigate through the decision process. My intention is to shed some light on the dark moments and bring hope to the reader. After all, blessings come in all shapes and sizes...*even three centimeters.*

CHAPTER 1

Trust and Believe in The Lord

I don't remember much about July 17, 2002, other than I met a man that day whose words changed my life as I once knew it. His words echoed in my head as if I had been told a very bad joke, yet those same words have since empowered me, lifting me higher than I ever would have imagined. How could those words change my quality of life for the better and bring me closer to my family, and my community?

You may have experienced hearing the same words yourself—you have breast cancer. To this day, they still sound like they belong to someone else and not me.

The day had started with a phone call, a wake-up call. I had been speeding down the road of life, when all of a sudden—boom! I was blindsided. I didn't see it coming, or maybe I did, but chose to ignore it. Breast cancer only happens to other women—women much older than I.

When I was 38, and our last child had just turned one, I noticed a lump in my left breast. Having had a benign cyst removed some nine years earlier in my right breast, I figured it was the same thing. Therefore, I didn't bother with it. I would forget about it until my son would sit on my lap at church and lean up against me. Feeling some minor discomfort, I would just reposition him and forget about it. I know, right now you're probably thinking how could I have just ignored it? I had my annual mammograms and my doctor knew about the lump. I was told that it was probably nothing and that I should just watch it. Watch it, what the heck does that mean?

I tried to ignore the lump, however, it reminded me of its presence when I laid on my stomach, or when I leaned my breast on something. But the mammogram said that it was nothing to be concerned about, and so I trusted technology over the knowledge of my body and continued to ignore it. I, like you, am busy. There's always tomorrow to worry about things, not today. I have cleaning to do, grocery shopping, kids' soccer practices, dinner to make, and a volunteer meeting to prepare for and attend. Maybe tomorrow I'll set up an appointment to get a second opinion, but not today. Yet, that tomorrow didn't happen. Instead, I washed clothes, checked my e-mail and worked outside in the yard. The lump had been there for a few years what difference would a few more make? Life continued to get in the way of taking care of myself, and the next thing I knew, I was busy working on my 25th year high school reunion. That's when I noticed that the lump seemed to have grown. Yet, I was too busy to schedule an appointment. The reunion was in five months, and I figured I'd make an appointment then.

When the reunion was over, I finally made an appointment with my doctor. He agreed that the lump had indeed grown and wanted me to get a breast ultrasound. It was the end of the school year and we had a vacation planned to Arizona a few days after school was out for the summer. I decided to wait until I got back from Arizona to have the ultrasound. After all, I didn't want bad news to ruin my vacation plans, just in case something was wrong. In the back of my mind I kept thinking:

> I'm young, strong, I don't smoke, and I exercise regularly. I have no family history of breast cancer; therefore, it couldn't be cancerous. It couldn't be.

The day after our flight back from Arizona, I went in to the hospital to have the lump in my breast checked out. After changing out of my blouse and into a gown, I was lead to a dimly lit room where I was asked to lay on a padded table. It had a clean white linen sheet placed on top of it. The ultrasound machine resembled the type of machine that I had seen before when I was pregnant. The technician placed the clear lubricating jelly on my left breast and began to move the scanning wand around. The difference between getting a breast ultrasound and an ultrasound when you're pregnant is that I was not able to see the screen. There were no little arms and legs, and no thump, thump, thump, of the baby's heartbeat to listen to. My eyes remained fixed on the ceiling as I prayed to God and Blessed Virgin Mary for help.

When the test was over, I was escorted to a small room where I was asked to wait. Now, I've learned a few things about technicians—they don't tell you much, and they're great at keeping secrets. You have to learn how to read between the lines of what they are saying and you have to learn how to read their facial expressions. Usually when the technicians are finished with their work, they will bring the film to the radiologist to read. Once the film has been read and the technician comes back into your room and says anything but, Okay, you're all done, it's not a good thing. When they tell you, Excuse me, I'll be right back, it's probably not a good thing. The technicians are pretty cautious about what they tell you, which is usually nothing.

In the meantime, you begin to talk to yourself because no one else is talking to you. You tell yourself that they must be really busy and that you'll be fine. Soon you'll be home to prepare meals, listen to kids play or argue, wash the dishes, and all the fun stuff you do on a daily basis.

As I sat there in the tiny dimly lit room, I noticed the pictures hanging on the wall I thought to myself, why did they choose that ugly picture? From there, I embarked on a conversation in my head that went something like this:

Maybe I'll read one of the magazines sitting on the table? No, at the moment, I'm really not interested in how the movie stars get their abs in shape. Something's telling me that I'm going to have much more real issues to deal with than my flabby stomach. Oh, maybe I'll get a little informed by reading one of the brochures on the other table. Let's see, What You Need to Know about Breast Cancer. I'm sorry, now my stomach, you know the flabby one, is turning upside down. I can't bring myself to read that either.

Finally, the concerned technician re-entered the room and asked if I had time for one more test. They'd like me to get a mammogram. Once again, I struck up a conversation in my head:

They'd? Who are they? How many people were looking at my ultrasound results? Why does everything have to be so secretive? It's my body. Will someone please tell me what's going on! Okay, I might as well get the mammogram since I'm here anyway.

When I was finished with the mammogram, there was more waiting. This time I thought that maybe I should read the brochure about breast cancer. After all, I was just reading. It's not like reading about it would actually give me breast cancer. It's funny but sometimes we're afraid to read about something that might concern us for fear that the truth will come out—the truth that we can't face just yet. However, the truth always comes out. The truth was there all along. It just took me a long time to face up to it. Once again, the technician came in to my room, but this time, with the radiologist.

They both agreed that I should set up an appointment as soon as possible for an MRI. An MRI is a magnetic resonance imaging machine. With the help of a dye that is injected intravenously, the MRI machine acts like a huge magnet looking for cancer cells. This machine can be quite successful in determining whether or not the breast cells in question are cancerous.

Upon my return to the hospital the following week, I prayed all the way as I drove what seemed like a very long fifteen minute trip. I prayed for God's love to be present in every nurse, technician, and doctor that I had to work with. Yes, I mean work with. Together, we were trying to get to the bottom of what my condition was. It's a win-win situation for everyone involved when you're all working toward the same goal. I was told that they would have to inject a dye in my arm. The dye would then travel through my breast and the cancer cells would be highlighted in the film. It was actually very fascinating to see modern technology at its best. First, I had to lie down on my stomach and place my breasts in a breast mold. My arms were placed down along my sides. With my forehead resting on a cushion and earphones on my ears, slowly the machine began to move and my body entered a chamber. I was told that the test would take twenty minutes, ten minutes before the dye was injected, and then ten minutes while the dye was circulating through my breasts. I was asked what music I wanted to listen to. I chose a smooth jazz station to calm my nerves.

While wrapped up in the MRI cocoon, I wondered where my thoughts would be for the next twenty minutes. At first I thought I could sleep and then wake up and realize that this had all been a dream, or a nightmare! However, that was impossible because the machine was too noisy. Out of boredom and fear, I chose to talk to myself again:

I know! I'll think about what I should make for dinner. Yeah, right! How about just pray and ask God for help. Okay, HELP! Dear Lord, please work through the staff here today. Please hold me and be present today. Please give me just what I need today. Dear Blessed Virgin Mary, please hold my hands and be with me today. Dear Guardian Angel please be with me and stay with me. Thank you all!

After what seemed like only five minutes, I heard the nurse say over the intercom that the test was over. Whew! I made it. Chalk it up to another one of those things that I am now an expert on, but didn't want to know about in the first place. When the nurse helped me off the table she said, "Well, I have some good news and some bad news. Which do you want to hear first?" "Ha, ha, this is a joke, right? You're kidding me," I said. "No," she said. "Okay, give me the bad news first."

"Well," she said, "Only half of the test worked, so you are going to have to come back tomorrow and do it again. We're going to have to shoot the dye back into your arm because that's the part of the test that didn't work and we don't know why."

I'll tell you why! The test didn't register because it was too crowded in the MRI chamber. Not only had I prayed and asked God, Blessed Virgin Mary, and my Guardian Angel to be present with me while getting the MRI, but I also prayed that both of my deceased grandmothers, my deceased mother-in-law, and anyone else in Heaven who likes me be present because I was afraid. I had relied on too many people to help me when all I really needed was one…God. It's no wonder the machine malfunctioned.

"Okay, so what's the good news," I asked? "The good news is that instead of the test taking twenty minutes, it's only going to take around ten minutes," the nurse said.

Wow, I thought, that's really good news—NOT! Oh well, next time I'm going to only ask for God to be present. Everyone else can wait in the waiting room!

I was back in the hospital two days later to get my second MRI. This time, the machine worked liked it was supposed to and I was done in no time. The MRI was quite amazing. It showed what the mammograms were not able to clearly pick up. Not only did I have one tumor (the one I felt), but there were two others below it lined up in a row like a constellation of stars. It was recommended that my next test be a breast biopsy.

Well by now I had been in and out of the hospital for about a month. With my birthday being right in the middle of the summer, you guessed it—the biopsy was scheduled on the day of my 43rd birthday. This was not exactly how I wanted to spend my birthday, having an ultrasound-guided needle biopsy, but I was left with no choice. It was going to be the last test and the icing on the cake. Happy birthday, Linda!

****

Two days later, I received a phone call from the nurse asking if my husband and I could come in later that evening to meet with a general surgeon. I knew this wasn't good news. Usually when you're fine, the nurse will just tell you over the phone. The receptionist may even leave a message on your voice mail or answering machine. However, when there's something wrong, they want you to come in. I was starting to get scared. I found I had to keep taking in deep breaths because my breathing was shallow.

Who me? It couldn't be! I don't smoke, and I can't say that I drink alcoholic beverages (does having a few glasses of wine or a beer every other month count?) I have no family history of breast cancer and I'm not overweight. Heck, I became a certified personal trainer just six months before my diagnosis, so what could this doctor actually be telling me? Oh, I'm sorry, I've made a mistake. My secretary got your chart mixed up with someone else. Sorry for the scare, Linda, but you're fine, our mistake.

There was a lot of silence in the car as my husband and I drove forty-five minutes to meet with the doctor—more silence in the waiting room. I glanced around the room to see the facial expressions of the other people waiting like we were. No one was smiling, but no one was crying either. I kept repeating in my head, whatever the outcome, I'm going to be fine because God is with me and I will live each day that I have on this earth for The Lord. I trust that He will help me find my purpose, and I believe that He will reveal more of Himself to me as long as I open my eyes and heart to the world in which I live.

"None of us lives for oneself, and no one dies for oneself. For if we live, we live for the Lord, and if we die, we die for the Lord; so then, whether we live or die, we are the Lord's. For this is why Christ died and came to life, that He might be Lord of both the dead and the living. Why then do you judge your brother? Or you, why do you look down on your brother? For we shall all stand before the judgment seat of God; for it is written: 'As I live, says the Lord, every knee shall bend before me, and every tongue shall give praise to God.' So [then] each of us shall give an account of himself [to God]." Romans 14: 7-12 [1]

Lesson #1: Trust And Believe In The Lord, Our God.

This lesson became my mantra. It helped me to stay calm. I would suggest that you create a mantra that works for you. Some examples might be: deep breath in, deep breath out; God is with me; take one step at a time;

Jesus loves me; one day at a time; or, I am strong and I can get through this for God is my light and my salvation.

When my name was called, my husband, Rich and I were escorted into a very plain looking room with gray walls, brown furniture, and white lights. There may have been other colors in the room, but gray, brown and white were the only colors I remember. The doctor and I had never met before and he was very curt and to the point. "Well, you have breast cancer," he said matter-of-factly, "And I don't think you're a candidate for a lumpectomy either. I think a mastectomy would be in your best interest." "Excuse me, I don't understand," I said. "Not only do I have breast cancer, but you're suggesting that I remove my breast as well?"

There was more silence as we walked out of his office. I now realized why no one was crying in the waiting room—they wait until they leave the building. As we drove in silence most of the way home, I kept looking down at my hands and feet. I couldn't look up because tears were running down my cheeks. Finally, Rich said, "Well, at least we know what we're dealing with." I wanted to scream, but nothing would come out. I wanted to sob, but I was too choked up. I wanted to sleep in the car, but my eyes were peeled wide open due to shock. I felt like I was in limbo. So this is what purgatory must feel like, I thought.

Growing up as a young Catholic schoolgirl in the 1960s, the nuns warned you about purgatory. In my head, I envisioned purgatory as a dark room with one window, and only one candle burning in the window. No other light and no amenities. Nothing. You just sit and wait by the window until an angel from heaven comes to get you. At that point, the angel would either bring you to Heaven or take you to hell. You would pray that you were good enough while on earth to enter Heaven's gates. Here I was in my own purgatory—waiting. Waiting to see if what I would experience would actually be hell on earth. I prayed to God and prayed the rosary that night. Whole-heartedly, I gave myself to God. As His child, I decided right then and there that I would listen to what God was trying to tell me. No longer would I go about my business here on earth without purpose. Finally, fatigued from worry, I fell asleep. I had put myself in God's hands.

The sun was peaking in my window the next morning bright and early. It was only 5:00 a.m. when I opened my eyes. I felt like I had been hit by a truck in the middle of the night. My sense of security had been stolen. It only took a few seconds to actually bring my life back into focus. At first, I thought it had been a dream. However, my feelings of loss were too real. Once the clouds vanished from my head, I decided that I was on a mission—a crusade to find the best doctors and get this cancer out of my body. I was angry. My body had betrayed me. It had let a foreign invader take up space in my precious breast. In order to deal with this, I chose to view the cancer as an enemy, my enemy. I would find the best doctor, the best hospital for me, and together we would declare war on the cancer. We were going to win! In my mind and in my heart, I was going to recruit every healthy cell that I had to fight this war. My war was in need of a general—someone to guide me…God, our Father, with the help of Jesus Christ, our Lord.

"Therefore, since we are surrounded by so great a cloud of witnesses, let us rid ourselves of every burden and sin that clings to us and persevere in running the race that lies before us while keeping our eyes fixed on Jesus, the leader and perfecter of faith. For the sake of the joy that lay before him he endured the cross, despising its shame, and has taken his seat at the right of the throne of God. Consider how he endured such opposition from sinners, in order that you may not grow weary and lose heart." Hebrews 12:1-3 [2]

The next step was to bring my diagnosis to someone I trusted, someone who could steer me in the right direction. My family doctor was just the man for the job. I called him to set up an appointment. I explained my situation to the nurse and she got me in to see him right away. It's funny how all of a sudden I was no longer a 43-year old wife and mother of three grammar school-aged children, but someone who had a *situation*. My doctor, a wonderful man, told me something that made the first step of the journey less painful. He said, "If you have to have breast cancer, this is the one that you would want to have." Right then and there, I knew I was going to make it.

Most people with a serious illness will view their life as BD (before diagnosis) and AD (after diagnosis). Something happens to you when you are faced with a life-threatening disease. Some people will look at the glass as half empty, others as half full. You can only guess which view you will have, but the truth is, you will never know until you are faced with an unfortunate situation—one that is *too adult*.

> *Too adult* – a situation that forces us to grow up
> faster than we had anticipated.

I found out that I was looking at life as half full, but only *half* full. This was when I realized that I had a second chance at life—a chance to do everything right that I had not done right before and make the glass completely full. After all, I am alive at this very moment, and I thank God for every day that I can say that. The house needs to be cleaned—so what, my son needs a story read to him first. It's amazing how your priorities change when you feel your life has been threatened. Don't focus on the glass as half empty. Look at your life right now as a chance to become stronger than ever before. Take a hard look at how you can make peace with yourself, your family, and your friends. Above all, thank God for a second chance to demonstrate just how precious you are.

****

My prayer for you: Dear God, please grant the reader the opportunity to put her trust in You. Through the support of others, please help her feel loved. Please heighten her awareness so that she knows You will be with her every step of the way. Please bless her mind, body and soul while You gently heal her. Amen.

CHAPTER TWO

Mind Games – Body vs. Spirit

The body: Stage 1 Infiltrating Ductal Carcinoma, DCIS, Invasive Lobular Carcinoma and LCIS. So what does all that mean? Well, let's just say that I had a garden variety of cancer going on. Infiltrating Ductal Carcinoma originates in the milk passage, breaks through the duct wall, then enters the fatty tissue of the breast and forms a hard lump. DCIS, or Ductal Carcinoma in Situ, is a noninvasive type of breast cancer. The cancer cells are in the milk duct and have not grown outside the duct, which is their site of origination. Sometimes these cells are referred to as pre-cancer cells. Invasive, or also known as Infiltrating Lobular Carcinoma, originates in the milk-producing glands. LCIS, or Lobular Carcinoma in Situ, refers to the abnormal cells within the lobule. It starts in the milk-producing glands and is usually not invasive. There are various stages of breast cancer depending on the size of the tumor and whether or not the cancer has spread.

Upon calling my OB/GYN and discussing my situation with her, I asked her for the name of a surgeon she trusted. Rich and I each came up with the name of one person we knew personally who had gone through a similar situation. We felt that these women would be good resources. We told our family and a few close friends of my situation, and that was it—the fewer people who knew about it, the better. I needed to keep my head clear to make the best decision possible for me. I didn't want to start hearing horror stories or everyone's advice. When we were done, we had at least three doctors to choose from. We made appointments to meet with them all within one week. We brought my films and a notebook filled with questions to each appointment. The notebook also contained a rating scale from 1 to 10, 10 being a perfect score. We based the following criteria on issues that we felt were important to us in making an educated decision:

- The doctor's personality—did we trust him/her?
- The doctor's advice.
- The hospital where the surgery would be performed.
- Our insurance.
- Referrals from trusted family and friends.
- The doctor's office and staff.
- The doctor's attention to detail.
- Whether or not convenience was important—doctor's office and hospital proximity to where we lived.
- Whether or not the doctor/surgeon sees patients on a daily basis—whether or not he/she is *in the trenches.*

Both Rich and I rated each doctor separately. We then totaled the categories and came up with an overall rating for each doctor. The doctor with the highest total would then perform the surgery. Two of the three doctor's totals were close. This system really helped us in making a decision—a decision that I have never regretted. Please see the chapter titled Questions To Think About located at the end of this book. This chapter can be used as a starting point to determine what's important to you. You may find that your decision will feel better if you can see it on paper. How would you handle a business transaction? Having information in writing will help keep the facts straight and your head clear.

Based upon our discussions with the surgeons, I was not a candidate for a lumpectomy. The MRI clearly showed that it would be in my best interest to have a mastectomy. We decided to have the surgery at our local hospital for the following reasons:

- The surgeon we met with went into greater detail than the other surgeons, and then explained why.
- He showed us how to read the MRI.
- His nurse was extremely helpful, nurturing and kind.
- I decided that I needed to be close to home.
- He sees patients on a regular basis.
- I felt comfortable with him, and therefore, trusted him.
- I was very comfortable with the hospital where the surgery would be performed, as well as their staff.

As I was thinking ahead, I knew that I would have to have chemotherapy treatment, as well. It made sense to be as close to home as possible. With a son in kindergarten, it was important to me to be able to drop him off at school, swing by the hospital's treatment pavilion, get treatment, and be home before my children walked in the door. I also knew that I needed to rely on family and friends to drive my children home from school and take me to the hospital for chemotherapy treatments. The closer I was to home, the easier life would be for everyone.

Once we made our decision with whom and where the surgery would be performed, we set up the appointment for surgery as soon as possible. For us, that was two weeks later. At that time, I actually began to get excited about doing something to eradicate the cancer from my body, but that was only half of the equation. I needed to talk to someone about keeping my faith strong. Not only was my body suffering, but my spirit was too.

The spirit: For the first time since I had become an adult, I was struggling with my inner strength—my faith. This was quite unusual for me for many reasons.

When I was eight months pregnant with my son, I was cleaning out one of our outside window wells. The cement wells are approximately three and a half feet deep and about four feet wide. The cement ledges surrounding the wells are approximately 1 foot wide. I had lowered an empty 30 gallon garbage can into it. As I stood on the cement ledge bent over with a broom in my right hand and a shovel in my left, I grabbed the leaves at the bottom of the well and placed them in the garbage can. This was the way I had always cleaned out the window wells and I felt very comfortable doing so. Walking slowly to the other side of the well, I lost my footing and began to fall into the well. My first thought was, oh my God, I'm falling. My second thought was, I can't because I'm pregnant. My reflexes kicked in. I dropped the broom and shovel and threw my arms out wide to the sides to grab on to something, anything, to prevent me from falling in. With my left hand reaching for the bricks outlining one of the living room windows, and my right hand trying to grab an evergreen bush, I felt the cement edge of the well scrape against my lower back. I was half in the well when all of a sudden, in a blink of an eye, I was standing back up on the cement ledge looking down into the well. It took a few seconds to wrap my mind around what had just happened before I realized it was a miracle. I slowly walked around the well and sat down on one of our patio chairs. Dumbfounded, I began feeling around my pregnant belly for any signs of distress from the baby. Luckily, the baby was fine and so was I, minus a few scratches on my left elbow from the bricks, a scratch on my right shoulder from the evergreen bush, and the scrape on my lower back from the window well. Either I had a guardian angel, or my baby (my son) did. Feeling a slight breeze around me, I looked up into the afternoon sky and felt giddy. I had been truly blessed. Why did this happen to me?

Perhaps so I may be witness and give testimony to God's power and to know that He is always with us. I slowly got up from the patio chair and went inside to tell my husband, Rich. "You're never going to believe what just happened," I began, and continued to tell him the whole story. At that moment, I knew the baby that was growing inside me was going to be named Michael. I chose to name him after the great archangel. Thinking that no one would believe me, other than Rich, I kept that miracle to myself for several years.

During my pregnancies, I had a heightened sense of awareness about my body. With each pregnancy, I dreamt of my children. I saw them all. Michael's image of blonde straight hair and blue eyes came to me when I was approximately four months pregnant with him. The only thing I remember from that dream was that I was pushing him in a stroller. The day after my dream, I approached my husband and said, "Well, if I'm correct again, this time we're having a boy."

Like as with Michael, God had given me the insight of seeing my two girls in my dreams during pregnancy, as well. I had a few dreams about Caitlin, my oldest. One time I saw her as a baby and someone else was caring for her. The other time, I saw her playing as a child of about twelve years in age. Her hair was no longer blonde, it was brown. Well, Caitlin was born a blonde, she did have someone care for her while I worked part-time, and her hair did turn a dishwater blonde/brown by the time she was in middle school. I only had one dream of Dana. I saw her during childbirth. She was smiling so big and I was smiling and everything was wonderful. Dana's sweet demeanor, always smiling, is still present today.

After all that I had witnessed during my pregnancies, and the guardian angel that caught my fall, I was upset with myself that I had doubts about my spirituality. I had become a doubting Thomas.

"But Thomas, one of the twelve, called Didymus, was not with them when Jesus came. So the other disciples were saying to him, "We have seen the Lord!" But he said to them, "Unless I see in His hands the imprint of the nails, and put my finger into the place of the nails, and put my hand into His side, I will not believe." After eight days His disciples were again inside, and Thomas with them. Jesus came, the doors having been shut, and stood in their midst and said, "Peace be with you." Then He said to Thomas, "Reach here with your finger, and see My hands; and reach here your hand and put it into My side; and do not be unbelieving, but believing." Thomas answered and said to Him, "My Lord and my God!" Jesus said to him, "Because you have seen Me, have you believed?" Blessed are they who did not see, and yet believed." John 20:24-29 [3]

Ask yourself this question: Have I become a doubting Thomas, or, am I more like Peter when he got out of the boat to meet Jesus as Jesus was walking on the water. Peter knew it was Jesus, but he let the wind distract him and he lost focus and began to sink.

*"At once [Jesus] spoke to them, "Take courage, it is I; * do not be afraid." Peter said to him in reply, "Lord, if it is you, command me to come to you on the water." He said, "Come." Peter got out of the boat and began to walk on the water toward Jesus. But when he saw how [strong] the wind was he became frightened; and, beginning to sink, he cried out, "Lord, save me!" Immediately Jesus stretched out His hand and caught him, and said to him, "O you of little faith, * why did you doubt?" Matthew 14:27-31* [4].

I made arrangements to meet with the pastor of our parish, Fr. Gerard. He was a slender, middle-age man, who was very approachable. Fr. Gerard had baptized Dana, had served on various committees with both my husband and I, and we had him over for dinner several times. Without hesitation, I picked up the phone to make an appointment with him. He detected anxiety in my voice when I spoke to him and gave me his undivided attention. Fr. Gerard cleared his calendar and I was able to meet with him the following day. Upon my visit with him, I was finally able to come to terms with my emotions. I cried, I vented my anger, and eventually, began making jokes about my situation.

"Hey," I told Fr. Gerard, "I can be the first one ready for church when my hair falls out since I won't have to spend time fixing it! We'll actually be on time now."

I also joked about taking up golf, and how I could always blame my prosthesis for getting in the way of a bad golf swing. Or, maybe I'll finally be able to swim since my prosthesis can float in a pool—it can keep me afloat. I was on a roll and actually found that by poking fun at myself, it made me feel in control. Feeling in control actually made the cancer seem less threatening. I was beginning to feel better already. We continued to talk about God and my relationship with God. It was so uplifting to realize that it's okay to be angry with God. Through Fr. Gerard, I learned that God wants us to come to Him with our problems. Well, I had some problems!

Sometimes God speaks quietly to us, and sometimes He speaks loud and clear. The point is, we need to be aware of God's presence in our lives every day and rely on Him for all things. We need to spend some time quieting ourselves, whether it's first thing in the morning, or just before bed, so that we can listen for God's voice. How do you listen for God's voice? Does it come by means of a conversation you've just had with someone? Do you hear God's voice in the laughter of children? Or, do you only hear God when you attend church? For me, sometimes it's a sharp, but sudden thought that may pop into my head and an instant sense of warmth that

I feel in my heart. I chose to seek out God's comfort and His grace as I depended on His strength to help win my battle against cancer.

While Paul was in Corinth, he wrote the following:

"Three times I begged the Lord about this, that it might leave me," but He said to me, "My grace is sufficient for you, for power is made perfect in weakness. I will rather boast most gladly of my weaknesses, in order that the power of Christ may dwell in me. Therefore, I am content with weaknesses, insults, hardships, persecutions, and constraints, for the sake of Christ; for when I am weak, then I am strong."—II Corinthians 12:8-10 [5]

For when I am weak, then I am strong—I love that phrase. What a beautiful thought it was, especially at that time. There will be days when you feel weak and it's okay because there will be days when you will feel strong.

Lesson #2: The Spirit Is Stronger Than The Body

Believe it and know that you can dig down deep inside and pull out your inner strength. It's there. Just ask and God will give you just what you need. As you grow in your faith through the grace of God and the breath of the Holy Spirit, your heart will be opened to a new beginning.

****

My prayer for you: Dear God, please help the reader find inner strength. Please use Your strength, oh Lord, to fill her with the Holy Spirit. Please grant her the opportunity to put her trust in You. Through the support of others, please help her feel that she is loved and that You are with her every step of the way. Amen.

CHAPTER THREE

God Sends Us Angels

God also demonstrated His presence through my friends. One group of women, in particular, comes to mind. I had the pleasure of meeting twice a month with a prayerful bunch of women looking to incorporate a deeper meaning of faith into their lives. My diagnosis came just a few days before one of our gatherings. Just as everyone was getting ready to go home, I asked them to keep me in their prayers. I spoke quietly about the results of my tests. It was the first time I was going public with my diagnosis. One of the women whom I had just met for the first time that day invited everyone to stand around me. As I sat in a chair, I felt truly blessed. Each woman had placed her hands on my shoulders and head. They asked the Lord to bless me and help me get through my fight with grace and support. It was hard not to cry and I felt embarrassed by my tears. They reassured me that I *should* cry. Their prayers touched my soul and the bottom of my heart so deeply that I felt like I had just fallen into a well—a well rich in love. It was the first of many beautiful experiences breast cancer had given me.

Another example of how God works through people on this Earth came the night before my surgery. My family had been invited to go to our close friend, Mary's, house for dinner. After dinner, Mary began to boil water for tea. The mood of the evening had been pleasant, but somber. We tiptoed around the subject of breast cancer and surgery. The kids had settled themselves in front of the television set as Mary and I sat down in the kitchen for tea. Just then, the doorbell rang. Strange, I thought. It's

9:00 p.m. at night. Who could be at their door? It was Della, another one of our good friends. She had heard about my surgery and wanted to wish me well. All of a sudden, the doorbell rang again and another friend walked into the kitchen while I was sipping tea. Walking quietly behind her, was another friend, and then another. By this time, (no, I've never admitted to being a rocket scientist) I realized what was happening and tears started streaming down my cheeks. Overcome with emotion, I began hugging everyone. I felt such gratitude that evening. These women and their families rallied around me. We all went outside and sat on the patio under the stars in the luminescence of candlelight. The night air was warm. A soft breeze swirled around us gently wrapping us together in a blanket of hope. We held hands and prayed fervently. We talked, laughed, and wiped tears from our eyes. Each woman had brought with them words of encouragement that were placed on paper neatly bundled in a beautiful white cloth bag. The bag had a white silk ribbon enclosure and was embroidered with a pink, blue, and green heart. I didn't read the contents of this precious bag until I got home. I quietly asked the kids to go to bed, told Rich that I would be upstairs shortly, and sat down to pour through my bag of prayers and well wishes. I read poetry, bible verses, and words of encouragement. The purpose of the prayer bag is to place your problems in the bag. Upon doing so, you place your trust in God by letting go of that problem. God will handle your problems if you allow Him to. *He will address your problem in His time, not yours.* Thus, patience is a virtue. I was grateful for that evening at Mary's house. I had prayed to God earlier that morning to give me just what I needed for that day. He did just that. He always does.

The following morning as I was getting ready to go to the hospital, the phone rang. "Good morning sunshine," chimed one of my best friends that I had known for several years. "What are you doing," she asked? "WHAT

AM I DOING?" I replied. "I'm getting ready to go to the hospital for surgery, what do you think?" I said sarcastically.

"The hospital, why?" she replied. "WHY?" I said. "Are you kidding me?" I said with a laugh. I told her why and she thought that I was having surgery on Friday, not Wednesday. It was a fluke that she had called early that morning. No, it was not a fluke. It was just what I needed that day. I had prayed, once more before I got out of bed, asking God to give me just what I needed. He did just that. He always does.

Lesson #3:
God Sends Us Angels When We Least Expect Them.

Somehow I knew that I was going to be fine. Although I was still a little nervous and trying not to have an anxiety attack, the phone call I received in the morning and the gathering the night before demonstrated first-hand how the power of God works in our lives with the people we love. I entered the hospital with a smile knowing that soon I would be on the road to recovery. After all, who needs two breasts, one can work just fine. One breast, or two, doesn't define who you are as a person. I'm still the same person, hopefully a little smarter, wiser, and more compassionate than before.

From the first person at the front desk to the last nurse I saw before I left the hospital the next day, everyone was very supportive. I felt I was truly in God's hands. The surgery went well and the sentinel-node biopsy that was performed came back clean. The cancer hadn't spread. I remember trying to wake up from the anesthesia in my hospital room after the surgery and my mom saying, "Linda, Linda, wake up. Your lymph nodes are clean." I opened my eyes realizing that my head was resting on my left side as if I wanted to cradle myself—cradle the side of the surgery and comfort the area where there used to be a breast. The position seemed to say, it's okay, the cancer cells are gone and you're going to be just fine. I opened my eyes again long enough to see my mom standing there, giving me the thumbs up. I closed my eyes. It's over, I thought. I thanked God and went back to sleep.

My stay in the hospital was short. I had learned from having three C-sections that I needed to be able to shower, eat my food, go to the bathroom on my own, and be fever-free before I could go home. I willed myself to do what I needed to do so that I could go home sooner than later. I wanted my own bed. I forced myself to eat the bland food, and I drank liquids constantly. When it was time to walk down the hall and shower, I was a bit apprehensive about getting undressed in front of the nurse. Yet, I didn't want to be alone with my new body either. When the shower was finished and I was back in my room, the nurse brought me in front of the mirror to show me how to change the bandage. Upon looking at my naked torso, I said, "Oh my God!" and quickly walked back to the hospital bed. I grabbed the vomit pan, but nothing happened. I was breathing heavy as Rich sat in the chair with a look of concern. The nurse approached and stood right in front of me. I looked up and she said, "Well, at least you're alive." Alive! She was right. I was alive and had a pretty good prognosis too. I got up and walked back over to the mirror for my lesson. That was the last time I felt sorry for myself. Now when I look at my scar, all I see is the beautiful work my surgeon did. I can honestly say I'm comfortable with my body. I have learned to love my body for what it is.

I was able to leave the hospital within 48 hours and was looking forward to a good night's sleep. There would be no more listening to the sounds of doors closing, the distant murmur of the nurses' station, and an impatient old man yelling down the hall for the nurse.

Another one of my very close friends, whom I had known for several years, had offered to watch the kids overnight the first night that I was home. She was truly a blessing. As much as I wanted to see my kids, I needed to rest. Later that night, Mary stopped by bearing gifts. As I was propped up in bed, she laid a pitcher of iced green tea, freshly brewed, that contained a hint of lemon. She gave me a little blue and white porcelain angel holding a prayer book that I put next to the little bluebird my mom had given me while I was in the hospital. My nightstand was beginning to look like a shrine adorned with holy cards, religious medals and books of inspiration. Mary sat at the edge of my bed, while Rich sat in a chair. We talked, discussed, and reminisced. When Mary was ready to leave, she assured me that she would be back tomorrow with a protein shake. Night had fallen. It had been hot for a couple of days and the windows had been shut so the air conditioning could be on. We weren't aware that the sounds outside had changed to signal the end of a challenging day. As she stood up, a lightning bug had appeared next to her head. It came out of nowhere and had startled her. "Do you want me to take it out of the house?" she said. "No," I said. "It's God's gift for me. It's my light. He's showing me the light. It's probably going to end up on the floor next to my bed sometime tonight, so leave it," I said. The funny thing is, we then commented on how we hadn't seen any lightning bugs yet, and since the house had been closed up, it was odd. Later that night, I woke up and laid there thinking of how blessed I was. I leaned over the nightstand to reach for my water, but the faint glow of a light on the ground caught my eye. There, on the floor, next to my headboard, was that little flash of light again. As I focused my eyes on the floor, I saw the lightning bug, shooting off rays of hope. The lightning bug was just where I thought it would be. God had given me just what I needed—He always does.

I began each day on my road to recovery taking baby steps. I didn't feel comfortable leaving the house while I had the drain attached to my body.

The drain was necessary for the removal of fluid that accumulates at the site where the breast was. There was a long tube that was inserted under the breast scar. This tube exited my body about four to six inches under my armpit. It then traveled downward into a drain, which resembled a small squeeze bottle. This bottle needed to be emptied about three times a day for a total of seven to ten days post-surgery. My job was to record the amount of fluid that accumulated in the bottle. It's important to stay on top of that job. You need to make sure that your fluid is decreasing in order to heal, and thus, allow the drain to be removed when it should be.

Because my dad knew I wasn't comfortable leaving the house, he came to the rescue. Like a true Italian, he took great joy in bringing me food. Every week for the next year he would go to his favorite Italian restaurant and bring back a container of soup. "Here, you need to eat this to get strong," he would tell me. He was right. I looked forward to my weekly visits with my dad. He would stay a little while and ask how the kids were doing. He became their biggest fan while attending their soccer, basketball, and baseball games. I thank God every day that I still have my parents in my life. As a result of my illness, my father and I became very close. I truly believe that the Lord works in mysterious ways.

The day of the Feast of the Assumption, I wanted to go to our Catholic church. Unfortunately, I was still attached to my new appendage—the drain! I had talked to my sister-in-law, Kathleen, earlier that morning. I was feeling a little down and she thought she would come over to cheer me up. I agreed. A visit from her would be great. As I was getting ready for my visit with Kathleen, the phone rang. It was Sister Betty calling to see how I was doing. She thought that I might be interested in receiving communion, and wanted to bring it to me. "How wonderful," I said. "My sister-in-law, Kathleen, is on her way over and so you can meet her."

What Sister Betty, Kathleen, and I shared that afternoon was a blessing. We sat in my living room, chatted, held hands, and prayed. I felt God's presence as Kathleen and I received communion from Sister Betty. Once again, God had given me just what I needed.

Two more angels and good friends played a role in my healing. They helped me with the uncomfortable task of changing my bandage. Believe it or not, people do want to help you. There are times when we need to ask for help from one another. God wants us to build community and communicate with others. Through our prayers, He brings people into our lives. Sometimes He does this for a short time and sometimes until the end of our life here on Earth.

****

Ten days later, my appointment with my surgeon warranted the removal of the drain. It was finally coming out and I was beginning to feel great. With the cancer gone, I had so much more energy than I remembered. I was ready to get out and get moving. When I came home, I decided to shower and get dressed up. Good-bye to my over-sized T-shirts I had worn during the last ten days to hide the drain. I was going to put a bra on for the first time since surgery. Since I did not have a prosthesis yet, I needed to be creative. My daughter, Dana, actually had a brilliant idea! "Mom," she said, "Why don't you take something and just stuff it in the left cup of your bra?" "I've got it! Dana you've just inspired me," I said. I had some old shoulder pads lying around from the 1980's. "I'll just try a few on for size," I said. I was still sore and wanted to wear something a little bigger. I found an old maternity bra that would work just fine. However, I needed a larger shirt, too, to hide the oversized bra. Boy, this was turning into a bigger deal than I had imagined. I was mumbling out loud, when Rich walked in to see how I was doing. When I told him I had nothing to wear, he said: "Oh that reminds me. I brought back a golf shirt from my business trip the other day. Why don't you try it on and see how it fits?" It fit perfectly and you couldn't tell what was underneath my shirt. I thanked God, and Rich. Once I was dressed, I stood in front of a mirror. Either I was going to be depressed because I looked ridiculous, or I might be pleasantly surprised. Not sure what I would see, or how I would feel, I closed my eyes. When I finally opened them, I was very surprised by my reaction. Not only did I feel whole again, I really looked it. I began to cry. Yes, there was light at the end of the tunnel. As I stood in front of the mirror crying at my new figure, I thought it might be therapeutic to record my emotional roller coaster ride on paper. I decided that I would go out and buy a very pretty journal.

A few days later, right in the middle of the afternoon, the doorbell rang unexpectedly. To my surprise there stood my friend, Nancy, with a plate full of brownies and a gift. It was nice to see her and I welcomed the visit. Just before she left, I opened her gift. I could not believe what I was looking at. It was the most beautiful journal I had ever seen. Tears came streaming down my face as I looked up at her remembering what I had said earlier that week. Thank you, Lord, once again!

****

My prayer for you: Dear God, please help guide the reader's friends in a way that shows love, not fear; guide them so that they reach out to her, not hold back and wait to be contacted; and, help engage her friends in prayer, not wait for others to do the praying. Amen.

CHAPTER FOUR

Post-Surgery Stretches

Lesson #4:
Post-Surgery Stretches, Exercises, And Massage (if applicable) Can Help You Feel Better And Recover Faster.

Each day I worked on regaining my full range of motion in my left arm. Full range of motion is the ability to move a part of your body, usually your arms and legs, as high as your joint potential allows you to. For example, you should be able to raise your arm straight up overhead. I received a video from my doctor demonstrating certain exercises necessary to accomplish this. Breast cancer can permanently change the way you take care of yourself. Most people want to regain control of their life. By eating nutritionally, getting enough sleep, proper exercise, and reducing your stress, you can. Exercise for cancer survivors is not only therapeutic, but very helpful for a positive recovery. As a certified personal trainer, I can't stress enough the benefits of exercise. As a cancer survivor, I found out first hand just how important exercise can be. This is your opportunity to make a positive lifestyle change. If possible, join a health club or a park district program. Some hospitals, and even churches, have programs for breast cancer survivors. Chemotherapy treatment, anti-cancer drugs, and radiation, can leave you feeling drained. Finding an exercise program that is convenient and fun will help you in so many ways. You may meet new people with whom you would like to socialize with outside of class. I suggest you check with your doctor to see if he/she knows of an exercise program that you can participate in. Also, check with your doctor to see if he/she has a post-operation exercise video or book that you can borrow. Ask your doctor if he/she has a handout that includes stretching exercises to regain your full range of motion. Make sure that you are under your doctor's care when attempting any type of stretching or exercise program.

Listed below in this chapter are a few lymph drainage exercises for the upper body as noted in the Cancer Exercise Specialist Study Guide[6] followed by some range of motion stretching exercises I used to help regain my complete range of motion. The range of motion exercises are from the American Cancer Society Exercises after Breast Cancer Surgery Fact Sheet that my doctor had provided for me in 2002. Please check with your doctor to make sure these exercises <u>are right for you</u>.

Important Tips: Do <u>not</u> perform pelvic tilts or basic modified abdominal crunches if you just had abdominal surgery in the case of a <u>TRAM-flap reconstructive surgery procedure</u>— (a portion of the abdominal tissue is used for breast reconstruction.) You should be at least 6 weeks post-op— (6 weeks after surgery) to perform pelvic tilts or abdominal crunches. However, everyone is different so please check with your doctor as to when he recommends you can begin such abdominal exercises.

Please stop any exercises if you feel swelling in the affected side/ arm of your surgery and notify your doctor. This could be a sign of lymphedema— *"swelling produced by an accumulation of lymph fluid in the tissue. For breast cancer patients, the swelling occurs in the arm of the affected side due to damage to the lymph vessels in the armpit area caused by the removal of the axillary lymph nodes or from radiation to that area."* Cancer Exercise Specialist Studyguide/Handbook. [6].

Basically, the fluid gets blocked and has nowhere to go so it is retained in the affected tissue. It's a buildup of protein-rich fluid that can accumulate in the arm, chest, or axillary region. I'm not telling you this to frighten you away from exercising because the benefits of exercise are amazing. I just want you to be aware and to let your doctor know if some swelling does occur. There are things to remedy the swelling like wearing a compression sleeve, massage, etc., that your doctor can help you with.

Check with your doctor to see if he/she knows of a trained lymphedema specialist that you can work with. You can also check with various health clubs to see if they have trainers on staff that know how to work with breast cancer patients. When you are cleared by your doctor, you may begin the following:

Lymph Drainage Exercises for the Upper Body:

Warm Up

Slowly warm the body up first. To do this, I recommend marching in place for about 3 to 5 minutes. While marching, add slow arm circles by placing your arms straight out to the side at shoulder height. First place the palms up, then turn your hands so that your palms are facing downward. Repeat slowly about 5 times in each direction. Bring your arms back down and change the march to knee lifts, hamstring curls, side steps, or anything that can get your heart rate up a bit. If you have a stationary bike, you can ride it for about 5 to 10 minutes, or alternate between marching and riding. If you have access to the outdoors, go for a 10 minute walk. However, I would not recommend riding an outdoor bicycle (non-stationary) just yet for fear that in case you fall you might injure your arm and/or your chest wall. Gage how you feel. If you don't have your energy back yet, then just walk around the house for 5 minutes to loosen up a bit. Eventually, you should start to feel stronger and more energetic.

When you are finished with your warm-up, check your heart rate. Make sure it resumes to a normal breathing rate so that you do not feel out of breath. If you feel out of breath, then walk around the room slowly until it returns to normal.

Once your heart rate has returned to normal (you are breathing normally) and you are no longer out of breath, lie down on a mat for deep abdominal breathing.

Deep Abdominal Breathing

Lie down on a mat on your back with your knees bent and feet flat on the floor. Arms are placed down by your sides. Keeping the small of your back snug up against the mat, take a deep breath in through your nose and blow out of your mouth slowly with pierced lips as if you were going to blow out candles. Repeat 5 times.

Continue with the exercises below:

Pelvic Tilts

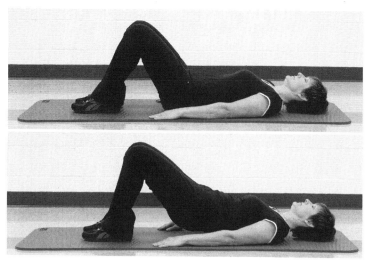

Begin pelvic tilts by lying on a mat on your back with your knees bent and your feet flat on the floor. Your head is down on the mat. Keep your chin up and your hands should be down by your sides and your low back should be snug on the mat. Now, slowly lift your hips and butt off the floor while keeping your head and shoulder blades on the mat. Your low back will lift up a bit. Squeeze your glutes (butt) and pause at the highest point of your lift for a few seconds. Then slowly bring your hips/butt back down to the mat to the starting position. Perform these pelvic tilts/lifts about 8 – 10 times.

Basic Modified Crunches

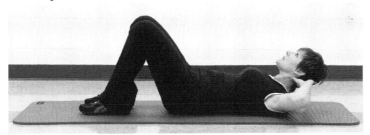

Continue lying on your back on the mat with your head down, feet flat, knees bent, and low back snug into the mat. Place your hands behind your head or across your chest if it is too uncomfortable for you to place your hands behind your head. Slowly lift your head, neck and shoulders (if possible) off the mat as you look straight up toward the ceiling counting to four as you lift. Hold that position for one second before slowly lowering back down to the mat. Maintain your gaze up toward the ceiling throughout the movement and keep your low back pulled into the mat. Don't pull on your neck to lift up. Use your abs to do the lifting even if it feels like you are not lifting very high at all. Keep your low back on the mat. Don't arch your back and don't forget to breathe out as you rise up. Continue the basic modified crunches for at least 8 – 10 repetitions.

By performing pelvic tilts and basic crunches, this will give the lymphatic system from the upper extremities a place to drain in to, thus decreasing the likelihood of lymphedema in the upper extremities. If you had a sentinel node biopsy, or if you have had any lymph nodes removed, you are at risk for lymphedema.

Neck Stretches

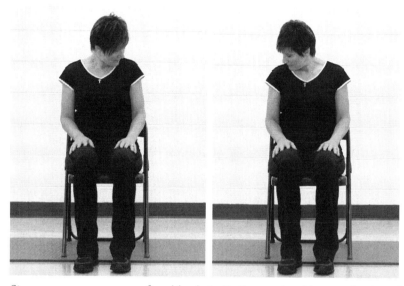

Sit on your mat or a comfortable chair. Roll your shoulders up, back and down to stretch them away from your ears. Next, gently turn your head to the right, back to center, then to the left and back to center (starting position). Exhale while moving your head to the right and left, inhale as you bring your head back to center. Continue the stretches by turning your head to the right and bring your chin down toward your right shoulder. Hold that stretch for 5 seconds before returning to the starting position with your head in the center. Slowly turn your head to the left and lower your chin toward your left shoulder. Hold for 5 seconds before returning your head to the starting position.

Shoulder Shrugs

Inhale while lifting your shoulders toward your ears, exhale and bring your shoulders back down. Repeat about 6 times.

Isometric Shoulder Blade Squeeze

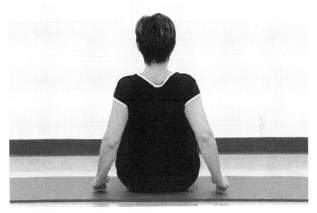

Exhale and slowly pull your shoulder blades down and squeeze them together. Hold that position for a few seconds then release the squeeze. Repeat about 8 times.

Isometric Chest Presses (prayer presses)

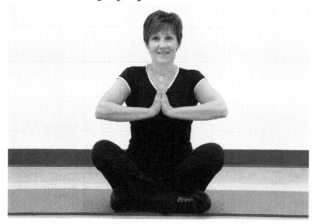

Place the palms of your hands together in front of your chest. Your elbows should be up with your forearms parallel to the floor (basically in a prayer position). Exhale and push the palms of your hands firmly together, hold for a few seconds, and then inhale as you release the tension in your hands. Repeat this 8 times.

Wrist Flexion

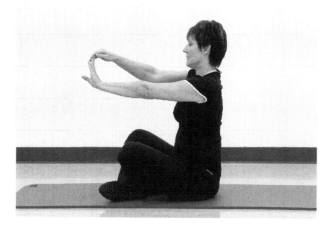

Bring your left arm straight out in front of you at shoulder height and position your hand as if you were telling someone to stop. With your right hand, grab your left fingers and, using gentle tension, slowly bend your wrist back a tad bit toward your forearm. This will be a very slight movement. Hold that position for 5 seconds then release. Repeat about 8 times with the left arm before switching arms.

Wrist Extension

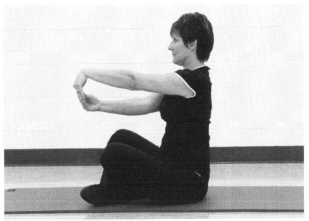

Bring your left arm straight out in front of you at shoulder height and position your hand with your fingers down. With your right hand, grab your left fingers and slowly bend your wrist down (opposite of wrist flexion) as if you were going to have someone kiss the top of your hand… just like in the old days!! This will be a very slight movement. Hold that position for 5 seconds then release. Repeat about 8 times with the left arm before switching arms.

Finger Stretches

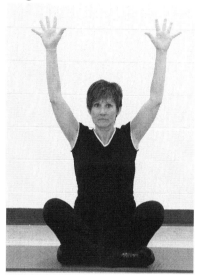 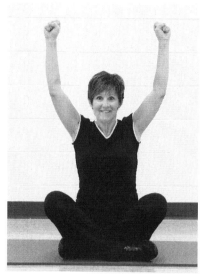

Lift your arms up overhead as high as you comfortably can. Open your hands wide by spreading your fingers apart. Then, close your hands into a fist. Repeat opening and closing your hands slowly about 8 times then lower your arms back down.

Range of Motion Exercises for the Upper Body:

Swinging Arm Circles

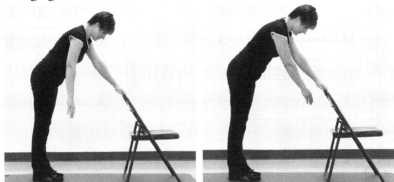

Hold on to the back of a sturdy chair or sturdy table that is waist high with one hand. While bending forward from your waist, let the other arm hang down and dangle. Slowly circle the arm in one direction about eight to ten revolutions then switch directions for about eight to ten revolutions. Switch arms and repeat the exercise with that arm.

Walking Your Fingers Up The Wall

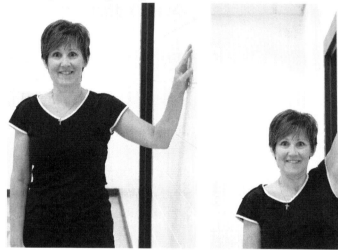

Stand sideways with your body of the affected range of motion side about twelve inches away from an empty wall. Slowly walk your fingers up the wall. Move in closer to the wall as you raise your arm further up the wall. Reach as high as you comfortably can then walk your fingers back down and step away from the wall to the starting position. Repeat this about eight times at least a few times per day until you regain all your range of motion. Using your other arm, walk your fingers up the wall the same way you did with the affected arm. Note how high that arm can reach and use that as a marker to help regain range of motion in the affected arm.

Doorframe Chest Opener

Stand in between the doorframe of any interior door in your house. Make sure the door will not swing back and close on you. Keep your fingers clear from the door jam. Keep your feet close together. Place your hands shoulder level on the inside of the doorframe. Now slowly lean forward slightly, holding on to the doorframe and keeping your feet in place. You will be off balance as the weight of your body moves forward. Hold that position and feel the stretch come across your chest and into your shoulders. Hold that pose for a few seconds and then return to the starting position. Repeat that stretch eight to ten more times.

Overhead Side Bends

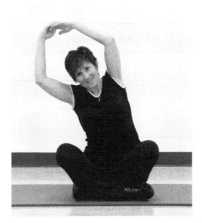

Depending on how you feel, you may do this stretch either seated or standing. If you are seated, sit with your feet flat. If you are standing, stand with your feet hips-width apart. Reach your arms up overhead. Clasp your hands together and slowly bend your waist to one side while keeping your hands clasped and arms stretched overhead. Bring your arms back to center over your head and slowly bend your waist to the other side bringing your arms into a side bend stretch to the other side. Bring your arms down before repeating this stretch about six to eight more times.

Overhead Arm Stretch/Tricep Stretch

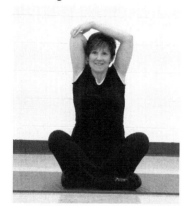

Depending on how you feel, you may do this stretch either seated or standing. If you are seated, sit with your feet flat. If you are standing, stand with your feet hips-width apart. Reach your arms up overhead. Bend the arm of the affected side at the elbow, dropping your hand and placing your palm on the back of your head. Place the hand of the other arm on that bent elbow of the affected side and slowly move the arm of the affected side back behind your head as far as you comfortably can without pulling or feeling pain on the affected side. Your hand of the affected side will move slightly down toward your shoulder blade. Hold that pose for a few seconds then switch arms. Bring your arms down and repeat about six to eight more times.

Supine Floor Stretch/Chest Opener

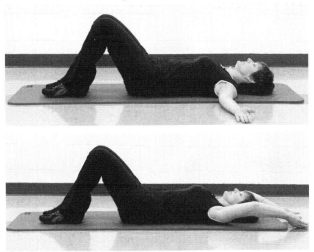

Lay down on your back on either a mat, comfortable rug, or your bed without pillows. Raise your arms up perpendicular to your body and then lay them down over your head. Keeping your arms to the floor or bed, slowly bring your arms away from your head forming a letter T. Your goal is to get your arms flat on the floor or bed. Hold that stretch for about ten seconds, making note as to how far away from your head you had to bring your arms down in order to get the arm completely on the floor or bed. Notice how different the affected arm is from your other arm. Repeat that stretch again, but this time, try to draw your shoulder blades together and open/stretch your chest. Repeat this exercise eight to ten times a few times a day until you feel you can get the affected arm in line with the other arm. Note: this is one exercise that you may need to do periodically for years to come as the body will continue to want to tighten up and draw the affected arm/arms in.

Broom Raise

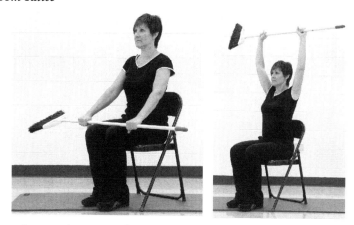

Depending on how you feel, you may do this stretch either seated or standing. If you are seated, sit with your feet flat. If you are standing, stand with your feet hips-width apart. Hold on to the handle of a broom with an overhand grip (your palms are facing your legs). Keep your arms shoulder-width apart. Begin with the broom resting on your thighs. Slowly bring your arms up until the broom is over your head and your arms are stretching back as far as you can. Slowly bring the broom down and back to the starting position. Repeat this exercise about eight to ten more times.

Horizontal Arm Stretch

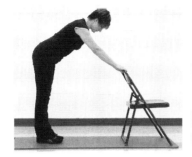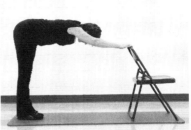

Face the back of a sturdy chair. Place your hands on top of the back of the chair. Slowly take a few steps backwards as you begin to bend from the waist. Keep your arms straight so that you don't hit your head on the back of the chair as you lower your head down while stepping away from the chair until your head is between your arms. Again, keep your arms straight. Try and not bend your elbows to do this exercise. Once you are in that position, hold your body there for a few seconds and feel the stretch. Then, slowly walk back up. Repeat this exercise at least eight to ten times a few times a day.

****

It took me about eight weeks to regain my range of motion performing those stretching exercises. I used the top shelve of our medicine cabinet to gauge my progress. My goal was to be able to reach it within eight weeks without bending my elbow and feeling discomfort. Walking my fingers up the wall a few times a day really helped. Of course, I waited until the drain was removed and I had permission from my doctor to begin. Range of motion exercises are an important part of any exercise program, but especially for breast cancer survivors. Improving your range of motion will not only help prevent problems such as frozen shoulder, but they will also help restore normal functional use of your arm(s), as well as, reduce the risk of lymphedema.

Another part of the healing process involves scar massage, especially if you choose not to have reconstructive surgery. Massaging the scar will help prevent the buildup of scar tissue. If possible, seek the help of a professional massage therapist, but check with your doctor first to see if you are a candidate for such massage. The massage therapist can help relax the muscle around the scar and assist in healing and regaining your full range of motion. A massage therapist may also show you how to massage the scar tissue yourself. I did have a friend who is a hand therapist and she advised that I use the tips of my fingers of the opposite hand and gently move those fingers in a circular motion up and down the scar tissue. I found it helpful to use a gentle lotion as I massaged my fingers clockwise and then counter-clockwise up and down the area of the scar. This massage technique became a part of my daily ritual for close to a year.

****

My prayer for you: Dear God, please help this beautiful woman heal internally and externally. May she continue to get stronger and view this time in her life as the beginning of a healthier and happier life. Amen.

CHAPTER FIVE

Managing ADL
(Activities of Daily Living)

During the eight weeks post-surgery, I was in the process of finding a medical oncologist. Although I had the surgery to remove my breast of cancer cells and my lymph nodes were clean, the doctors still believed that chemotherapy treatment and radiation would be necessary. I met with three different oncologists from three different hospitals. Each one had a different treatment in mind. Once again, I prayed for God's help. I was assuming that every doctor had my best interest in mind; at least I would hope so. However, medicine is also a business and it was helpful for me to view it that way when making my decision. Finally, a very good friend who is a doctor, pointed out that I should take advantage of all the advances medicine has made. Since two of the three medical oncologists suggested four treatments instead of six, and two of the three (although different oncologists) suggested radiation, I decided to go with the majority opinion. The medical oncologist I chose also was part of the same network of doctors that had performed my surgery. It made perfect sense for me to continue to stay in my insurance network.

Once that decision was made, I then needed to arrange my *activities of daily living*, or ADL, schedule. For some people who work full-time, this could mean you may have to schedule time off for your treatment. Yet, I know of other women who never missed a day of work. I found it helpful to schedule my chemotherapy treatments on Friday. This way, I had my family home with me on the weekends. Talk with your employer about the possibility of flexibility. Check with your family about how they perceive your battle with cancer. How involved in the treatment process do they want to be, and how involved do you want them to be? Keep lines of communication open. Cancer does not only affect the person who is sick, it affects family, friends, and in some cases, your community. The best laid plans can sometimes go awry when it comes to the human body. Think through each of the days of the week and write down what you do on those days. Check to see where you can obtain help from family, friends, neighbors, and/or support groups. One of the ways I was able to reduce my stress level was on commute time. Since I worked part-time near my home, I chose an oncology facility that was approximately fifteen minutes away from my home. You have to keep in mind that you will be spending a lot of time traveling back and forth in between follow-up doctor's visits, and the actual treatments themselves. Therefore, where do you spend the majority of your time? Will you be going to work in a city that has a medical facility nearby where you can schedule your treatments and follow-up visits? Or, do you work out in the suburbs and would rather take advantage of the location of a suburban hospital?

As I looked at my calendar, I realized another reason why choosing a facility close to my home was important. It would allow me the opportunity to be there for my children when they came home from school. By reaching out to my neighbors, I arranged for my children to be driven to and from school. My energy could then be used to repair my body, instead of driving around. Our church community has a group of women volunteers called the Kitchen Angels. These women cook and deliver meals to the homes of people in need. The Kitchen Angels offered to help me by preparing and delivering dinner three days a week beginning the first week of my chemotherapy treatment, and twice a week the following week. On the third week, I was on my own, which was what I had agreed to My treatments were every three weeks, and I needed to be back on my feet by that third week anyway. Therefore, meals from the Kitchen Angels were not necessary by week number three. On the days that they were scheduled to bring my family and I dinner, their delicious meals were such a welcome sight, especially on the days when I felt very tired. Contact your local church to see if they have such a group. Some churches offer a volunteer program called Meals on Wheels. If your church doesn't offer such a service, then ask them if they know of another church or support group that does. There are people out there who want nothing more than to volunteer their time and talent to help those in need. Reach out to them. After all, God wants us to help one another and experience community.

Ask and it will be given to you; seek and you will find; knock and the door will be opened to you." Matthew 7:7 [7].

Luke 11:9 repeats this bible verse from Matthew's Gospel by saying,

"So I say to you, ask, and it will be given to you; seek, and you will find; knock, and it will be opened to you." [8].

The Lord works in mysterious ways and with the help of special people. Open your heart to The Lord and let Him show you His love in ways you can't imagine. Give your extended family, friends, and neighbors the opportunity to help you and your loved ones at home. Pray to God every day and give Him thanks and praise. He has been patiently waiting for you. God will help you through this time of pain with the help of other people. It may not be the exact way you would like Him to and it may not be at the very moment you want Him to, but He will help you.

Lesson #5:
Manage Your Life With The Help Of Family, Friends, Neighbors And/Or Support Groups.

Once I had my medical oncologist, rides for my children, and meals from the Kitchen Angels all set up, I was able to focus on getting physically stronger before I began chemotherapy treatment. The longest any oncologist would allow me to wait was eight weeks post-surgery. They wanted to begin treatment as soon as possible, but I wanted to regain my strength first so that chemo wouldn't knock me down too bad. Seeing that I had a mastectomy and my lymph nodes were clean, the medical oncologist I chose to go to for my treatment granted my wish and allowed me the eight weeks before I began chemotherapy to focus on getting my body stronger.

Soon, I began enjoying early morning bike rides, pedaling through the woods of a nearby bike trail for about a total of forty-five minutes round trip. Since I had lost a bit of strength in my left arm (the side of my mastectomy), I began lifting three pound weights, which was light compared to the eight pounds I was able to lift prior to my surgery. It's important that you start out light and slowly work your way up in weight to avoid lymphedema. I made it a point to incorporate either walking or bike riding at least four to five times a week and light strength training once or twice a week. I performed one exercise per major muscle group and repeated that exercise for twelve repetitions; simply, lunges and squats for my legs, back extensions and one-arm rows for my back, various sit-ups and crunches for my abdominals, front and lateral raises for my shoulders, and bicep curls and tricep extensions for my arms. *Refer to the last chapter of this book for these exercises.* My experience and my body taught me that it was best not to perform push-ups and chest flyes just yet. Therefore, I did not do any exercises for my chest. There would be plenty of time after my chemotherapy and radiation was over to focus on a stronger strength training/cardio program. Breast cancer survivors, who have had lymph nodes removed, are at greater risk for developing lymphedema (a swelling of the lymph nodes that create the retention of protein-rich fluid in the affected area). I must reiterate, it is important to ease into any exercise/stretching program. Listen to your body and start with light weights (1, 2, or 3 lbs.) at first.

Having taken the eight weeks to eat smarter, sleep more, and exercise slowly, I felt I had done all I could do to prepare my body for chemotherapy. Chemotherapy, as with any drug, can create weight gain. It is important to try and maintain a healthy weight for your body frame. Therefore, take care of yourself. Eat smarter, sleep well, and exercise by walking and/or doing light meditation.

Praying had also taken on a major role in preparing my mind for what lie ahead. A healthy mind and body work together in sync. God was my answer to help get my head in the game. He is always there waiting for you to come to Him.

"Therefore I say to you, all things for which you pray and ask, believe that you have received them, and they will be granted you." Mark 11:24 [9].

I prayed to God several times a day and asked Him to give me strength and courage. I asked Him to encompass the medical staff with compassion and patience. I prayed for all the people who were suffering in the hospital, for the people who were homeless, abused, or at war. I begged God to hear the cries of His people throughout the world and to be there for them, to give them a sense of peace, and comfort them with a blanket of hope. Cancer is bigger than you and me. It's everywhere in this world and affects everyone in some way. I encourage you to pray to Our Heavenly Father for whatever tugs at your heartstrings and gives you a sense of uncertainty.

God has a plan for us all. It is not up to us to decide when that plan shall be revealed. Therefore, live each day to your fullest. Trust in God for He will show you the way through His son, Jesus. Nothing and no one on this Earth can take His place, so don't give anyone or anything else that power.

****

My *prayer for you*: Dear God, please grant this beautiful woman the courage to reach out to others. At this humbling time in her life, may she be surrounded by caring people who embrace her as they offer her their support. May she feel comforted in knowing that You are always with her and Your good works are evident in those around her. Let her see the image of Jesus in all those who surround her and care for her. Most of all, Dear God, let her feel Your love as her blanket of hope. Amen.

CHAPTER SIX

Dear Journal

Lesson #6:
Keeping A Journal Can Help You Come To Terms With Life.

August 18, 2002

Dear Journal,

I will begin my journal not at the beginning of my diagnosis, but yesterday, August 17th. It was the second day of my neighbor's garage sale. For every year we have lived on our block, we have always participated in it. When the kids were babies we would set up a playpen outside in the shade. As they got older, they started selling their own toys and books. They loved talking with potential customers. Sometimes, they would take the money they made and turn around and buy something from my neighbor. Eventually, we put the kids in charge of checkout. They learned how to add and keep records of our sales. It became my girls' favorite job at the garage sale. This year, the garage sale was a blessing as it helped keep their minds busy while I was still struggling with external healing.

August 22, 2002

Dear Journal,

As if I don't have enough on my mind already, let's add about 50 more reasons to be freaked out…50 small, but annoying black and yellow reasons. It's a good thing I know a wonderful exterminator. My bedroom door is now shut with a towel under the door to make sure the bees don't get out. Thank goodness Rich is out of town because I'm going to have to spend the night on the couch. As it turns out, there's a bees' nest in our built-in wall air conditioner. I've been watching the bees swarming outside my bedroom window near the air conditioner unit since June. Why I decided to have the nest destroyed in August, I'll never know. Because of this, the bees' entrance to the nest was crippled and they needed to get out somehow. Into my room they flew, and flew, and flew everywhere. My room looked like something out of a horror movie. Hopefully, they will no longer be taking up residence in our house tomorrow. After all, they're not even paying rent!

August 23, 2002
Dear Journal,
I had to open the door to my bedroom. I just had to. I had to see what was going on. Slowly and carefully I peeked in. The room was quiet. On the floor next to the French doors, were approximately one hundred dead bees. According to the exterminator, whatever bees are left in the nest after he sprayed should be dead within 24 hours. As a precaution, I decided to close up the air conditioner unit with a sheet and secure it with duct tape.

Yesterday's bee episode put a damper on things. However, I realized that I'm stronger than I thought. If I was able to run out of my room as quickly as I did, I surely should be able to drive. I know the doctor is concerned about my ability to react quickly while driving, but he should have seen me react yesterday!

August 24, 2002
Dear Journal,
It's 1:30 a.m. and I am jolted out of bed by Rich swatting at something. The poor guy got stung, not once, but three times in his foot. I felt so bad for him, but happy that it wasn't me. I didn't tell him that my mom had advised me to make my bed for fear that a bee would end up in it. Of

course I thought, "What would be the chance of that happening?" So I left my bed unmade. I wasn't very good at listening to my mother when I was younger, maybe I will now. Sorry Rich!

August 25, 2002
Dear Journal,
Today is Sunday. I'm aware of God's presence in all things, and keeping a journal has helped me get a handle on my life. I pray that I may see the goodness in all things, and I pray for a sense of peace throughout this day.

Each day, after my shower, I walk my fingers up the wall. The shower helps to warm the muscles up a bit, making it easier to stretch a little farther and reach a little higher each time I perform the exercise. I'm grateful that each day is an improvement, perhaps a bit small, but I do see an improvement. It's hard to imagine having complete full range of motion after experiencing such tightness under my left arm. Yet, I am determined and convinced that I will regain the ability to lift my left arm as high as my right within eight weeks, if not sooner.

September 2, 2002
Dear Journal,
I'm taking this day a little slower than yesterday, as yesterday was not a good day. It was one of those days when I should have listened to my body. I've been pushing myself a lot and was tired. Rich took the kids to the Cubs game so I could rest. Instead of napping, I thought a little trip to the store wouldn't hurt. However, I had to drive Rich's car because he had mine. His car is a little larger than mine.

Maybe I should have someone take me to the store, I thought. No, I'm really tired and I should just rest, I thought some more. Nonsense! I'm just getting a few things. I'll be back before you know it, and then I'll rest.

So I left. As I was backing out of the driveway very slowly, I didn't see the little car that was parked directly behind our driveway. BAM! I tapped it. I couldn't believe it. How could I have been so careless? The car belonged to our *new* neighbor's brother. *Our new neighbor!* What a way to meet them. Uh, excuse me I'm your neighbor across the street. Welcome to the neighborhood and, uh, by the way, I just hit your car.

Fortunately, they were very understanding. Unfortunately, there was just enough damage that the door to his foreign car would have to be replaced. The only damage to Rich's car was some of the paint on his bumper had been rubbed off. I was in hot water. I hope that the Cubs won to soften the blow!

September 30, 2002
Dear Journal,

As I await chemotherapy treatment, I know that it will be through my pain and sorrow that all kinds of beautiful feelings will prevail. I will now face my chemo with a much more uplifted spirit. By preparing my mind, I am able to prepare my body.

Side note: Cancer treatment can be a mind game. You really have to lift your chin up, hold your head high, and believe that YOU CAN DO THIS! Read books and articles that you find uplifting. Do not read anything that is going to bring you down. Get your head into what your body will be experiencing. God can help. Pray to Him to help you find your inner strength. Draw on His and look to God for comfort.

Next, if you have time between your surgery and the first day of treatment, check with your doctor to see if he thinks it's advisable to exercise. If so, practice very slow, relaxing movements. Go for walks and do your stretches. This may help you feel stronger prior to treatment. This also means eating right and getting plenty of sleep. Read food labels so that you are only eating healthy foods. Go to the library and find books on nutrition. Now is the time to educate yourself so that from here on out, you can become the strongest, healthiest person you've ever been. Breathing and meditation helped keep my mind focused on daily blessings. Our bodies respond to our feelings and what we believe in our minds. Therefore, feed your mind first. Surround yourself with positive people. Read inspirational articles and books. You'll find that in no time you will feel better about yourself, and you will be aiding your body on the road to recovery. Hang in there and believe in yourself. You are stronger than you think. Thank God for that!

October 3, 2002

Dear Journal,

Tomorrow I begin my chemotherapy treatments, the first of four. God gave me another gift today…a hummingbird. I don't recall ever seeing one around here. Yet, I've seen one now three times. The bird is an iridescent turquoise blue. I feel blessed in another way today too. One of the hospitals that I have met with took a look at my x-rays and called with the good news. They believe that my right breast looks free from disease. They also feel that although radiation to the chest wall would be beneficial, it may not necessarily be something that I need to do.

October 4, 2002 – 3:30 p.m.

Dear Journal,

The day started out gloomy with rain. At times, I felt as though it's Heaven's tears streaming down in place of my own. Chocked up with a lump in my throat, I couldn't cry. My throat was dry. Very much aware of the watch on my arm, I kept checking the time…three more hours before I begin my treatment; then, two more hours until chemo; then again,

30 minutes and counting. Finally, when Michael went off to afternoon kindergarten, I wept.

Once I arrived at the treatment pavilion, I found the nurses were very sympathetic. My good friend, Justina, took me to my first treatment. I needed to be with someone who was available in the afternoon and who would have a very calming, reassuring demeanor. I was nervous. Within the hour I realized I had nothing to be afraid of. Inserting the chemotherapy intravenously in my arm went better than I had imagined. A television set was on, but I couldn't tell you what was on the screen. The conversation was sporadic and light as I drank my water. I had to keep believing that this process was going to help me. I know the anti-nausea medication the nurse had administered was working. I prayed and prayed. I needed to know that both God and our Blessed Virgin Mary were with me. I pacified myself by envisioning that God was holding my arm—the one that chemo was being shot into.

We finished treatment with 15 minutes to spare. Our children's school is just a five-minute ride from the hospital treatment pavilion. As Justina and I sat in her car outside of school waiting for the children to be released, she hugged me and said, "You did it! One down and three more to go! See, piece of cake. You can do this." As the children entered the car, one-by-one, they told me stories of how their classmates were praying for me. Dana, my ten-year old, had given me a bunch of cards that all the children in her class had made for me. It was very comforting to know that for the next several months, I would have a lot of people praying for me. With the support of family and friends, I can set up carpools to allow myself time to rest in the afternoon, just before the kids get home from school. I need to conserve my energy so I can fight the negative effects of chemo and any residual cancer cells. Blessings do come in all shapes and sizes. This time it was a very large Catholic school and church community.

Once we got home, the focus was on the kids. I wanted that focus. I didn't want to think about myself. When they were finished with their homework, I walked outside and felt the warm autumn breeze. There was even a warm smell in the air too. I began to get giddy thinking I can do this. I can get treatments and not fall apart. I'll order a pizza for dinner, get the kids ready for bed, and then pray and read for inspiration. Simple!

October 4, 2002 – 9:00 p.m.
Dear Journal,
It's now 9:00 p.m. and not one problem. I am tired, but I was tired from the onset of the day. I hope that tomorrow is tolerable. The Zofran (anti-nausea medication) is going to be taken twice a day, every 12 hours, for another two days.

October 5, 2002
Dear Journal,
Today is Saturday and we're enjoying a day filled with sunshine, blue sky, and cool breezes…just the right ingredients for a fall day. I am feeling fine. The Zofran is doing its job. I am a little tired, but that's because I didn't sleep well last night. I think I slept for a total of four hours. My goal each day will be to try and take an afternoon nap, drink water religiously, and read inspirational material.

October 6, 2002
Dear Journal,
Okay, I'm not feeling too energetic today. I've decided to stay in bed this morning and let the sun beat down on my face through the window as my family goes off to church. As I lay here, I'm very much aware of the sounds outside—birds, cars, planes, the gentle breeze blowing in the trees, and the distant sounds of conversation. Perhaps this journey is one of self-renewal. Perhaps this time in my life of being forced to slow down

will show me a new way of existence, or even a purpose. Maybe even a life that opens doors to allow more people in, and allows me to be in more peoples' lives.

As I lay here, I decide to watch TV. A Catholic station was broadcasting a mass. Digesting each word that the priest is saying, I feel a sense of peace as I relax. For the first time in months, I feel the weight of the world being lifted off my shoulders. Praying, I begin to experience the joy that comes after the pain. The joy you feel when you give yourself completely to God. God has put me on this earth, and only God will bring me home to Heaven when my purpose is done. Gazing out the windows of the French doors of my bedroom, I experience a beautiful feeling of surrender as I look up into the blue sky. What a comforting feeling of knowing that the One Most High was in charge and not me. Closing my eyes I feel tears swell up inside. All the years of trying to find myself and questioning my place in life didn't matter anymore. Maybe this is what it feels like to grow spiritually and emotionally. My second chance at life was just that, a second chance to do life right.

October 10, 2002

Dear Journal,

Well, its 11:00 p.m. This is my first night without Rich since chemo began. Around 6:00 p.m., I felt like I wanted to cry. I was able to push my feelings aside when our dinner was delivered. When 7:30 p.m. came, and I couldn't push my feelings aside, I called a friend who I knew would understand. As my voice began to speak, I could hear the sound of my voice straining to remain calm and unemotional. I needed to say that I was sick and tired of feeling sick and tired. My friend listened and offered to bring a movie over to cheer me up. With the kids in bed, I settled in to watch a touching story about an angel named Michael. When the movie was over and I finally decided to turn in for the night, I discovered that my own little angel named Michael had positioned himself comfortably in my bed and was fast asleep. I gently picked him up and carried him into his own bed. Bending down to kiss him on his tiny warm cheek, he smelled nice and clean and looked so peaceful. I stood over him for a few minutes just wondering what I did to deserve such beautiful children.

October 11, 2002

Dear Journal,

I'm trying to take it easy because I'm not feeling too good. I've played I SPY with Michael and have read one book to him. Right now, he's playing with his cars. He told me I could take a break from reading. Nice kid! Actually, I'd like to take a break from a headache I have right now. According to one of the medical oncologists in my doctor's practice, I should continue to experience tingling and discomfort in my head for another couple of days since my hair is getting ready to fall out. However, I have broken out with acne cysts on my scalp, which is uncommon, and it really hurts. Last night, I couldn't sleep because my head kept hurting. Acetaminophen helped, but not for long. Tonight, I've taken two Ibuprofen tablets and I hope it works. I hope God answers my prayer.

October 12, 2002

Dear Journal,

No sleep again. My head still hurts. I'm mad and disappointed. It hurts to touch it.

October 13, 2002

Dear Journal,

My head still hurts. God, where are you? Why is this not going away?

October 14, 2002

Dear Journal,

My head is still broken out and it hurts tremendously. Why am I experiencing such pain? Of all the people I've talked to who have undergone chemotherapy treatment, and unfortunately, there have been a handful, NOT ONE has ever experienced what I'm experiencing. I wonder if this is normal? I know there are a lot of side effects, but this is ridiculous!

October 15, 2002

Dear Journal,

I'm calling the doctor today to make an appointment because this is not right. I must have an infection going on under my scalp or something. I hope to get in to see her right away.

October 16, 2002

Dear Journal,

Relief is finally here—it's called an antibiotic. I do have some type of secondary infection on my head. I should have called the doctor sooner. I didn't realize that my condition was not a real common side effect. I hope to get some sleep tonight. Right now, the kids are playing a song on the keyboard they just made up. Actually, it's really good. My hair hasn't fallen out yet, but it will. Only God knows that I really do fear losing my hair. I'm afraid that I'm going to look like a man. However, maybe my infection is a blessing in disguise because at this point, I've been too uncomfortable to worry about how I'm going to look. Actually, right now, I don't care. I just want my head to feel better. I never thought I'd say this, but I'll be glad when my hair falls out. I'm sick of how my scalp is. So instead of freaking out about losing my hair, I'm going to welcome a nice clean, bald, but healthy head. Maybe it won't be so bad. I can wear pretty scarves and after all, I do have a wig that looks just like my real hair. Just think of all the fun I could have. For a different look, I can wear my wig backwards!

October 17, 2002

Dear Journal,

Today I received a surprise visit from a fellow breast cancer survivor. She brought over some beautiful scarves. I'm so grateful that she did. Blessed is a better word! I thank God, again, for all the goodness that has come out of experiencing breast cancer…seriously. The support we are receiving from this community is incredible!

October 20, 2002

Dear Journal,

Last night was the first night I could sleep without taking acetaminophen or ibuprofen. Thank God! Today my hair has started to fall out. A few strands here and there. I'm going to put some in this journal as a reminder of what my hair looks like. I understand that it could come back a different texture or color. Good, because I never really liked my hair anyway! I've heard of people losing their hair every which way. Some people just go and shave it off first. Because of my curious nature, I'm going to let it fall out however it wants to. It should be interesting. My energy level is normal and so I was able to make a real nice dinner. We attended the 6:00 p.m. mass and even my dad joined us. He has been going with us just about every Sunday since the end of July. I love that he comes with us. I was even able to go to Caitlin's outdoor soccer game today.

October 24, 2002

Dear Journal,

My hair is almost gone! It's been coming out in the shower and when I brush it. The shower is too messy. It falls out all over my body and is a pain to get off. I've since decided to wash my hair, or what's left of it, in the kitchen sink. This way, it will be caught in the drain. Yesterday was not that great of a day. It's very hard to deal with hair loss. I feel sorry for men. At least I know mine will grow back. Rich keeps telling me, "Now you know how I feel!" Poor guy, actually I do. I thought it would be a good idea to rent a movie and watch it in the afternoon. Woohoo! I never do things like that. I feel like I'm on vacation. However, I picked the wrong move to watch. The main character was dying, so I cried and cried. Actually, I needed to cry. Today I feel better. Tomorrow is my second treatment and I'm feeling okay with it. I prayed to Blessed Virgin Mary today. Every time I do, I always feel much better.

Sunday, October 27, 2002

Dear Journal,

After receiving my second treatment, I feel the same. Yesterday wasn't bad. Today I'm a lot more tired than I have been. I occasionally feel aches and pains. I'm trying to drink a lot of water. I know it helps. Rich has been a tremendous help. He has had to do a lot of shopping and has become the soccer mom. My stomach has been a little upset. Maybe tomorrow will be better.

Side note: After that journal entry, I started spending about 30 minutes a day doing light yoga, walking, stretching and very low intensity aerobic exercise. Each day I made sure that I took the time to rest. I was able to do light housekeeping. My family agreed that they all needed to pitch in and help more than they have. Again, with this newfound freedom, I was able to relax and read more. I was even able to rent and watch a movie in the afternoon without feeling guilty! By the time the kids came home from school, relaxation time was over. There was homework to do, soccer practices, and meals to contend with.

One of the most helpful things that my friends of our parish did was to bring our family dinners. The first week after treatment, dinner arrived at our doorstep, hot and delicious, around 6:00 p.m. Monday through Friday. The second week after treatment, dinner came three times that week. By the time the third week came, we were on our own. I can't tell you how grateful we were to receive meals. The time it takes to plan, cook, and clean-up after dinner is incredible. This way, I was able to focus on getting stronger and giving the kids the attention they needed. Sure, there were times when I didn't feel good. When that happened, I would lay down for a while. Then, I would get up and get moving. The best advice I could give anyone going through this is to listen to your body.

I made sure that I drank as much water as possible. I wanted these drugs to pass quickly through my body. Drinking lots of fluids helps tremendously, as well as deep breathing and light exercise. You want to get the oxygen and blood flowing throughout your body. With each treatment session, this becomes more apparent. With each treatment session, you may feel a little weaker. I found that I had to forego working with weights because the chemo was just breaking all my cells down. I didn't want to believe that I would lose muscular strength, but I did. Yoga became a very important component to maintaining whatever muscular strength and endurance I had.

November 19, 2002

Dear Journal,

I can't sleep. It's 1:30 a.m. I'm hungry and a little nauseous. I feel like I'm pregnant! Cereal, here I come. Now I can see how some people can actually gain weight while undergoing chemo. I hope this doesn't become a habit.

It's now 2:00 a.m. and once again, I lay awake in silent prayer. My thoughts turned my gaze to the window next to my bed. I was looking in the sky for the presence of God. As I was searching for the moon, it occurred to me that the light I was looking for was actually inside of me. I didn't need to go looking for signs. God is with us and in all of us. We need to look inside ourselves to see His light.

The following day, I received a surprise visit from another one of my close friends from my childhood who had just returned from a trip to Europe and was passing through on her way back home to New York. We only had about an hour, and as good friends do, tried to pack that hour with as much talking as we could. I was always the queen of gab, but this time I just wanted to listen. Just before she left, she pulled a tiny white satin bag out of her purse. "Here, this is for you," she said. "I bought it in Paris where I lit a million candles for you in every church I passed."

Inside the bag was a beautiful 14K gold charm of Our Lady, Blessed Mary. Also in the bag, was a holy card with a medal of Notre Dame molded inside the holy card. But what I really cherished was the rosary that lay on the bottom of the satin bag. The beads were like black iridescent crystals. "The rosary was blessed by a priest from one of the churches I went to," she beamed.

When our visit was over, I thanked God for her and each and every one of my family and friends that I consider to be precious gifts.

December 12, 2002
Dear Journal,

The Christmas season is upon us and I'm having a hard time feeling enthusiastic. Help! I'm tired of being tired. As I lay in bed, my safe haven, I start to daydream. I think back to a time in my life that was very simple—a time when simplicity and innocence went hand-in-hand. My thoughts bring me back to age eleven when my biggest chore was pushing my baby sister in a buggy up and down our block. With my transistor radio in hand, I would flip back and forth between the only two cool music stations there were. I remember standing beside my next door neighbor while he pitched a rubber ball over and over again into a self-painted strike zone on the bricks of the front of his house. I can still feel the gentle, warm breeze of the willow trees swaying overhead. If I close my eyes, I can hear the shhhing sound of the leaves playing with the branches of this great big canopy of a tree. Memories also bring me to the distant sound of an aluminum pop can being kicked down the alley as my brother successfully comes out of hiding to declare himself the winner of "kick-the-can".

Gone are the days of lying in the grass on hot summer days, starring up at the clouds. The cool grass would give relief from the hot breath of the summer wind. The billowing white clouds would become our entertainment of animal objects. Not once did I ever think I'd see God there. But somewhere up there, He was. Creating wonderful memories of my childhood—playing running bases, ghost in the graveyard, red light/green light and lemonade stands. Gone are the days of carrying around my transistor radio and choreographing dance routines to the latest in pop music. It had been years since my dolls had tea parties, or my brother's miniature toy cars were parked in a make-shift dirt driveway formed by small stones.

My mind continues to drift to the time when all the girls on our block would build forts in the snow to hide during snowball fights. We also used the snow to build the outline of our future houses. Standing about three feet tall, the snow walls became a bedroom, living room, and kitchen on our front lawns. The best part was the ability to create anything I wanted out of the snow. My prize creation was a dressing room table that held a snow-molded telephone on top. The phone would come in handy if I needed to call one of my childhood movie star idols. My friends and I would try and imagine what life would be like when we were older…we had no idea.

I'm much older now, life is not as simple, and my days of innocence are long gone. Life is just *too adult* right now. Thank God my last treatment is over, however, the fight is not yet finished. Once again, I will enter the breast cancer boxing ring in January when I begin radiation.

****

My prayer for you: Dear God, please help the reader find comfort in expression through journaling. May she feel relief from the burden of this disease through the power of the pen and may she also become closer to you, Oh Lord, for the rest of the days of her life. Amen.

CHAPTER SEVEN

Your Journal

Lesson #7: Keeping A Journal Is A Great Way To Express Your Feelings And To Feel In Control.

Today I'm feeling:_____

Because: _____

_____

_____

_____

Blessings are all around you. What did you experience today that you might consider a blessing in disguise? _____

_____

_____

_____

Think positively and find a bright side to this day. Today, I thank God that: _____

_____

_____

_____

Sometimes there will be days when you are not able to find a bright side or blessing. That's ok. Rest, stay hydrated, eat well, pray, and look for a bright side tomorrow. Today is one of those days because:

_____

_____

Write down 1 thing that could have made this day better. How might you be able to improve upon that tomorrow?

_____

_____

_____

Questions or concerns that I have today that I may want to share with my family and/or doctor: _____

_____

_____

_____

_____

Is there anything tugging at your heart today? Any thoughts you would like to journal for future reference?

_____

_____

_____

_____

_____

****

My prayer for you: Dear God, please guide the hand of the writer so that she can feel at peace through her words, thoughts, and prayers. Have her come to know Your goodness throughout this process of journal entries. May she come to know Your mercy, love and grace all the days of her life. Amen

CHAPTER EIGHT

A Visit From Childhood Friends

Of all the blessings I have, I can't help but mention my childhood friends. These special ladies know everything about me, and I know the same about them. I tend to break down each decade of my life as a different period of my growth. Each decade they were there. We became the support network for each other. Sometimes we cried together, laughed together, went out dancing together, traveled together, stood up in each other's weddings, ate together, or watched movies together. This time was no different. The support network continued and continued to grow stronger. One of my close friends lives about two hours away by car. We spoke on the phone quite often so when she decided to make the drive and come over to spend the day with me, I was thrilled. Knowing that my hair was gone, and whether or not it was out of respect for me, or she was just being silly, she knocked on my door wearing a scarf. What a true friend! She said that if we were going to go out for lunch together, we might as well look the same.

Lesson #8:
Childhood Friendships Are Reflections Of Our Past.

Mindful of the days of our childhood, I reminded her of the poem we wrote together when we were thirteen years old. One of the verses mentions that "We have so many items the same." I just looked at her and laughed. That day, our "items the same" were our scarves. It was nice to be out…to feel normal again. If anyone was going to look at me strangely or with pity while we dined, they would be looking at two of us.

We were two friends wearing scarves and enjoying the day together. Later that afternoon, a few more friends joined us. When they saw us wearing scarves, they too, wanted to wear one. Well, they had come to the right place. I had scarves in every color. While wearing our scarves, we sat around the kitchen table doing what we do best—eating, laughing, and conversing. We telephoned my brother, who lives across the street from me, and asked him to come over with his camera to take pictures of us. The loss of my hair was becoming everyone's entertainment as my brother walked in wearing a bandana on his head. I never imagined we would have had as much fun as we did. My friends and I laid in a circle on the floor with our scarf heads next to one another as my brother took pictures while standing over us. When my brother left, I asked my friends if they wanted to see my wig. I will never forget their response. "WHAT! You have a wig? You mean to tell us that you have chosen to wear this silly scarf all day when you have a wig?" First of all, I didn't ask anyone to wear the scarves, and secondly, I thought that's what friends are supposed to do…support each other. Verbally cornered against a wall, I was demanded to produce the wig. I was busted. "Why," they asked, "Do you not wear your wig?" "Actually," I replied, "I think the scarves are so much more comfortable. Besides, I like to change my look every day," I added. I excused myself and came back into the room wearing the wig. They all applauded. By this time, we were already feeling pretty silly. I proceeded to show them how versatile a wig can be. You can wear it backwards, I demonstrated. Or, you can wear it like this, as I showed them how it would look worn sideways.

The next thing I knew, my wig was no longer on my head, but on each one of my friends' heads. It was like a storybook fable where each woman was trying it on for the perfect fit. As the wig was passed from head-to-head, it started to take on a life of its own. First, it resembled something that looked like a squirrel sitting on top of a gray head of curls; next, a raccoon hat; and lastly, a shiny black motorcycle helmet as the wig was clearly too large for the head it was on. While they were all having fun, this meant that my bald head had become exposed. Fortunately, who else but with old friends can you make yourself completely vulnerable. We laughed until we cried. I felt like a princess as each one of my stepsisters tried on my wig. Instead of going to a ball, we were having one!

****

My prayer for you: Dear God, please help the reader embrace her lifelong friendships as the true blessings they are. Lifelong friendships don't necessarily have to be someone she has known since childhood, but can be someone she has just met that she feels a real kinship toward. These people come into our lives when we need them most and will stay with us. Please, Lord, grant this reader the opportunity to know what a lifelong friendship is and the wisdom to be able to recognize it. Amen.

CHAPTER NINE

God's Presence

I found myself anxious the day of my third treatment. For some reason, I couldn't settle myself down. Maybe I knew what was coming. I was white as a ghost when I walked in the door of the treatment pavilion. I didn't feel that good either. My head wasn't in the game, and my body felt it. My friend, Carole, who is a doctor, was not working that day and was able to drive me to my third chemotherapy treatment. She sat next to me as I nervously tapped my water bottle with my left hand. My right hand didn't move while the nurse tried to get the intravenous line going in my arm. "I have good veins," I told Carole. "Usually the nurse finds it quickly and the line goes in right away," I added. Why was today different? As I sat there hardly breathing for fear that I would feel pain, I realized that I was probably a bit dehydrated. Darn, I thought. I blew it. Dehydration is the key to feeling better. It also helps when you have to get your blood drawn, or are having a needle placed intravenously. At that point, I just chalked it up to experience. What else could I do? I made a mental note that the next time, which will be the last time I receive my chemotherapy treatment, I would come fully hydrated. Eventually, the nurse was able to do her job successfully, and the treatment began.

Later that evening, right after dinner, I excused myself and made the climb up the stairs to my bedroom. I wasn't feeling that great, and figured that I would be better off resting. When I was getting undressed, I discovered a leaf in my shirt. "Where the heck did that come from?" I said out loud. It must have fallen from the tree in our patio when I came home from my treatment. Instantly, I thought of God because He knows that this particular leaf was from my favorite tree. I smiled as I got down under the covers and thought about all the little things that He had given me. At 9:00 p.m. the girls were getting ready for bed. They came upstairs with ginger ale for my stomach. Dana thought it would be a good idea if we all prayed so that I could feel better soon. The girls climbed on my bed and we all held hands as we prayed. Their little hands were soft and warm. I instantly felt comforted. First, we prayed the Lord's Prayer, and then, The Hail Mary. We made up our own prayers, too. While discussing all the blessings and gifts that are in each one of our lives, we remembered the lightning bug, the hummingbirds, and the leaf. We just couldn't think of what the significance was of the bees that had nested in my bedroom air conditioner unit. What was that all about? We thought that God was telling us either to *bee aware, or bee careful.* Well, if you're *aware* of bees in your bedroom, surely you'll *bee* careful I thought, so, no, that's not it. Then it occurred to me. As I held up the leaf that was adorning my nightstand, I said, "Bees, leaves—bee-leaf—**Believe**!" Maybe He was just telling me to believe in Him. Maybe I should just relax and allow God to take control. Thanking the girls for my ginger ale, hugs, and words of wisdom, I told them that it was time for bed. I knew that tomorrow would be a better day and the sooner I went to sleep, the faster tomorrow would come. Getting into a comfortable spot, I closed my eyes as my hand held on tightly to the leaf.

****

By the time Thanksgiving was over, I had only one more treatment. It took me a little bit longer to get my energy back after my third treatment. How frustrating. I knew that I was going to need help with Christmas. I just didn't have the energy to shop or decorate. Fortunately, my husband is an excellent shopper and loves to do it. The children were more than happy to decorate the house. Due to the fact that I didn't have the energy to do anything, I gave in and lowered my expectations of how the decorating should be done. Upon doing so, I found great pleasure in letting the kids decorate the house however they wanted. The funny thing was that they really did a very good job. Wow, why had I not let go of control years ago?

Maybe it was because I knew the fourth treatment was my last, or maybe because I knew the procedures of the treatment process, I was actually looking forward to going to chemo. I didn't flinch when it was time to administer the drug into my arm, and I had made sure that I drank plenty of water beforehand. This time my companion was my husband, Rich. He sat there quietly reading his newspaper, while I was chatting with the staff. Just before we were finished, one of the staff members approached me with a gift. Since it was my last treatment, they handed me a basket that had an adorable cloth lining in it. I recognized the basket immediately since I used to sell that very type of basket. It was a Longaberger basket with a cloth liner covered in pink ribbons representing breast cancer.

Lesson #9:
Relax And Look For God's Presence In Your Life.

Evidently, a former patient bought several of these baskets and donated them to the treatment pavilion to give out as a token of hope. Wow, I thought, what a wonderful surprise…what a wonderful gift! We said our goodbyes, and Rich and I went home. As we drove in silence most of the way home, I kept looking down at my hands and feet. I couldn't look up because tears were running down my cheeks. This time the car ride was different than that long ride home from the doctor's office when we were first given my diagnosis. This time as I sat starring at my hands and feet, my eyes glazed at the basket of hope between them. This time my tears were of joy and relief knowing that hope was more than just an object—hope was a blessing.

My chemotherapy treatment experience had brought me to a new place in life. I felt I was no longer the same person I was several months ago and probably never will be. Now, there were many unanswered questions I never had before. What do I do now? What is my purpose in life? How do I feel physically, emotionally, and spiritually? Can my family fill in for me when I'm too tired to carry on activities of daily living? Who am I? Am I strong or weak? Can I humbly accept help from those who want to help? Am I the type of person who can hold my head up high in public with no hair on my head, eyebrows and eyelashes, knowing that I am being looked at differently? Will I be able to help others in a similar situation? Will God always be with me as much as He is now? How do I take this negative situation and turn it into a positive?

What I *do* know is that I am loved by so many people. I have been blessed. God does love me and I have so much to give. I will continue to live with compassion one day at a time. I will do a better job looking for the good in people and trust that the Holy Spirit will dwell inside me and help me to do so. I will continue to pray to God asking Him for His guidance, and I will seek Him out in everything I do.

"Come to me, all you who labor and are burdened, and I will give you rest. Take my yoke upon you and learn from me, for I am meek and humble of heart; and you will find rest for yourselves. For my yoke is easy, and my burden light." Matthew 11:28-30 [10].

****

When the day came to begin radiation, the sun was sparkling on the newly fallen snow. The air was cold and crisp, but the sun felt warm. I proudly sat in the waiting room among the other people for I, too, was now a cancer survivor. Slowly scanning the room's motionless faces, I soon realized that I was the youngest patient and most of their eyes were looking at me with sympathy. I didn't want their sympathy. Instead, I wanted to be an example of a cancer survivor with a very bright future. I wanted God's presence to be evident. Since my son was in afternoon kindergarten, I conveniently scheduled my 25 radiation appointments for 1:15 p.m. Every afternoon, Monday through Friday, I would drop him off at school, stop by the treatment pavilion for radiation, and be on my way within fifteen minutes. Each time I walked into the waiting room, I always had a smile on my face. I hoped that my smile would somehow lessen the anguish of the sad eyes that looked back. My goal was to be a constant light in the room and to breathe hope into the air.

****

When my treatments were finally over, my medical oncologist strongly recommended that I take Tamoxifen, a daily oral pill, for five years. If my body could tolerate this pill, it would help keep the cancer from returning by 50%. I agreed, and fortunately, tolerated it very well. I'm pretty confident that exercising at least 4 to 5 times a week helped to keep my weight under control and the feel good endorphins going strong! It was easy for me to settle back into a content life of teaching group fitness classes, personal training sessions, family, friends, and daily worship. Hungry for a richer life of spirituality, I attended a one-day seminar that focused on healing your body and soul. The day provided an opportunity of reflection for women with cancer. It was just what I needed to continue my spiritual journey and to feel God's presence. A beautiful card was given to each of us that read:

"When you come to the edge of all the light you know and are about to step off into the darkness of the unknown, *faith* is knowing one of two things will happen: there will be something solid on which to stand, or you will be given wings to fly." The author of this remarkable passage is unknown, and yet embraces the soul of each and every one of us just like a loving parent.

Hebrews 11:1; 11:6-7; 11:11 Now Faith is the substance of things hoped for, the evidence of things not seen. But without faith it is impossible to please Him: for He that cometh to God must believe that He is, and that He is a rewarder of them that diligently seek Him. By faith Noah, being warned of God of things not seen as yet, moved with fear, prepared an ark to the saving of his house; by which he condemned the world, and became heir of the righteousness which is by faith. Through faith also Sarah herself received strength to conceive seed, and was delivered of a child when she was past age, because she judged him faithful who had promised. [11]

We created touchstones on beautiful cards with a satin ribbon running through it. These touchstones were our personal written words that helped us individually learn how to heal. My touchstone words were: the birds, the moon, the firefly, the leaf, the bees, and the sun. We placed our touchstones in the center of the room which was surrounded by candles burning bright. The room was filled with the sweet smell of incense and flowers. Emotions were expressed on paper with watercolor paints. We were asked to choose two colors. One color would represent how we felt when we were first diagnosed, and the other would represent how we were feeling now. By placing both colors in the center of a white piece of construction paper, we let our paint run from one end to the other, keeping within the circle that had been sketched in the center of the construction paper. What emerged was a portrayal of our inner soul—a symbol representing the depth of our pain. Whether we felt joy, pain, happiness, anger, or peace, we were healing! My symbol looked like a turquoise quarter moon, shy of shining in its full glory in front of an orange sun as brilliant as a glowing sunset. I came home that day feeling a little more complete, a little more at peace, and a little stronger.

Within three months, I had regained enough strength to lift five pounds comfortably. Spring had arrived and I was eager to take my exercise routine outdoors. Just about every morning, weather permitting, I would ride my bike to a nearby bike trail and follow the path for about five miles. It became my therapy. What a wonderful way to begin each day— wrapped up in nature like a big quilted blanket. Trees, birds, squirrels, deer, and plants would make up each patch of the quilt, with God sewing every stitch tightly together. My senses were alive with the sounds of gentle blowing leaves and the chatter of birds. The change of the season was in the air—the smell of rain and the decay of leaves, the moisture evaporating from the pavement, and the crisp north winds filled my senses with a deeper appreciation for creation. Witnessing the beauty that God has created for us to enjoy, enabled me to fill my heart and soul with an inner peace. I felt the wind blowing around me, the rain gently touching my hot skin, and the heat exuding from my body, as I peddled hard to get strong. But what I really felt was *alive!* The solitude I experienced in the woods on the bike trail, gave me every opportunity to feel thankful, hopeful, and free, as I rode in a joyful silent prayer. God's presence is good!

****

My prayer for you: Dear God, please grant the reader the gift of inner peace. Help her to slow down and recognize all things pleasing to her. Put a smile on her face and a song in her heart today and all days that she turns to You for help and guidance. Shower Your grace upon her so that she is brought into the light of a brilliant sunset. Carry her away from the edge of despair and into a sea of hope, taking note of all that is good around her. Inner peace is only a prayer away. Amen.

CHAPTER TEN

Leading By Example

Each day I felt a little stronger and a little more fortunate. Although I was forced to temporarily slow down, I was almost relieved. It gave me the opportunity to take notice of the little things in life. These blessings or gifts are around us every day, but most of us don't take the time to look for them. I had learned to thank God for everything He had given me, especially my parents. My mother was instrumental in laying down my spiritual foundation. She taught me to acknowledge God and give Him thanks and praise. She was raised a Baptist in a small Indiana town. Her church and the Bible were a very important part of her life growing up. She carried her faith with her in everything she did and she passed that faith on to me. You can say God has always been a part of my life, but I let life get in the way of being close to God. It wasn't until my life was threatened that I woke up to the realization that if I wanted to feel peace and happiness, I would have to make God a larger part of my life. It was with the grace of God, that I was given a second chance and I was determined to make the best of it.

In early May, I received a call from our church pastor. He had invited me to be one of the speakers on Mother's Day. I was truly honored. During the past several years, we all had been enlightened by the words of some truly remarkable women. Now, he was asking me to join them. I was so thrilled that I said yes immediately. Of course, no sooner did I hang up the phone I realized accepting this honor meant that I had to write a speech. Oh no, I thought. What the heck am I going to say?

I immediately went to my journal and began an outline. I worked on that outline for one week. At least he had given me some time to prepare. Thank God! I wrote and re-wrote my speech every day, each day changing just a little. Finally, at 5:00 a.m., the morning of Mother's Day, I was back at the computer for one final draft.

"Good morning, I began. My name is Linda Hillsman and I am honored to be here. My husband, Rich, and I have been blessed with three children—Caitlin is 12; Dana is 10; and, Michael is 6. They all attend the day school and we are very proud of them. We moved into our home 13 years ago this weekend, and have been active parishioners ever since.

When Fr. Gerard called and asked if I would speak today, I was thrilled and a little nervous. Those who know me will agree I tend to have a lot to say!

When our children were babies, people would comment on how early they started talking. I would ask them, "Why are you surprised? Just take a look at who their mother is."

Motherhood is a journey that is constantly changing direction. At one point, we are the student, learning from our mothers—our role models. Then, upon the birth of our first child, we become the teacher until we get home from the hospital and realize that we really don't know what we are doing and so we're back to being the student again. You might also say that we are like a shepherd taking care of his flock. Just like in today's gospel according to John, Jesus said, "I am the good shepherd. A good shepherd lays down his life for the sheep."

I think we do that as mothers. We put the needs of our children before our own. My mother-in-law and mother are two examples of that love.

When I married my husband, Rich, his mother became a second mother to me. She was a great inspiration. She was involved in her community, her church, and her family. She loved people and had a great sense of humor. She was never judgmental and had a way of making people feel special. Every now and then I would call her for advice. If I told her of an upsetting situation, she would simply reply, "Linda, just ignore it!" If I told her someone was getting under my skin, she would say, "Linda, just ignore him or her." But what if that SOMEONE was my husband? What do you think she would say? Probably, just ignore him! I often said, "If I could be half the woman she was, I'd be doing great." Every mother has a gift that they give to their children. The gift I received from my mother-in-law was to lead by example.

My own mother inspired me in different ways. She made it her priority every day to clean the house, do laundry, prepare three balanced meals, and give us just enough activities to keep us busy. In other words, out of trouble. She would lead my brother, sisters, and I on expeditions in our backyard looking for rabbit tracks in the snow. "Maybe you'll find some deer prints if you look hard enough," she would say. Then she would excuse herself to go make us some hot chocolate. What we didn't realize was that growing up on the southwest side of Chicago with fenced-in yards, was highly unlikely that we would find deer prints in our yard. She was firm, fair, creative, an excellent cook, and quoted the Bible quite often. But what I take with me on my journey into motherhood from my mother was her love for God.

Last summer, when I was diagnosed with breast cancer, my first reaction was to pray and have a big, long conversation with God. At a time when your faith can become challenged, it was my comfort with prayer that I thank my mother for. She showed me how to ask God for help and to ask the Blessed Virgin Mary for her grace. My role as a mother took on a deeper meaning. I reached out to my children and embraced them in a different light. I saw each child as an angel utilizing their special talents to keep the household running smoothly. The movie title, "Angels in the Outfield" comes to mind.

Caitlin stepped up to the place and became the team manager. She helped with meals, homework, and laundry. She was experiencing first hand some of the responsibilities of motherhood. "Do you like being a mother?" she would ask. Although she didn't appreciate the responsibilities, she hadn't yet experienced the love that comes with it. "Yes," I told her, "very much."

Dana was our coach—my spiritual advisor! We would sit on my bed, hold hands and pray together. We would then share with each other what God had told us in our silent prayer. "God told me that you are going to be ok," she would say. "I know, He told me that too," I would add.

Michael, my son, was the pitcher. He would intuitively feel what I need and then throw a curve ball to get me laughing. Or, he'd throw a fastball to get me out of bed so that I had to see what he was doing right at that very second. "Michael, mommy's not feeling good and she needs to lie down." I would say. "But, momma, you have to see this cool building I made. You'll feel better after you see it," he would add. Or, "Momma, you have to see this tower I built out of the whole bag of marshmallows! I KNOW you'll feel better after you see this!" He was usually right. But my favorite pitch was Michael's change-up. He would tiptoe in our room while I was resting, and set a glass of water down on my nightstand. He really knew just what I needed.

Rich became the best catcher any team could wish for. He caught all of Michael's fastballs; he caught flak from the girls; and caught all my ups and downs. He's had quite a year. Even the Cubs want to sign him up!

In closing, I think the greatest gift I hope my children will receive from me is the gift of love. Our family has been truly blessed. Our parish has been blessed, too. We are a church of compassionate families and the home to so many mothers who lead by example every day. So on this Mother's Day, let us all give thanks for our mothers—our role models, and the women of this parish community.

Thank you and Happy Mother's Day!"

Lesson #10: Lead By Example

****

My prayer for you: Dear God, please give the reader the support that is needed from family to help fight this disease. Please bless the woman who is battling cancer right now. Help her feel empowered so that she can continue to make positive steps in a faith-filled journey. Give her the grace to lead by example. Amen.

CHAPTER ELEVEN

One Year Later

Before I knew it, June had arrived and marked my one-year anniversary from the time I began testing for breast cancer. It was also the time for my first mammogram with only one breast. I've had at least half a dozen of them before, but this time it would be different. This time I would be skeptical of the technician's facial expressions. This time I would only have one breast to be examined...hmmm, does this mean I qualify for a discount? However, some things would be the same. I would still ask God to be with me and pray that the test comes out clean. I would still occupy my mind with an endless to-do- list to pass away the time. I would still sit there on a cold chair wearing a paper thin robe, flipping through magazines while trying to breathe normally. Breathe, deep breath in, slow lightly forced breath out through my pursed lips I would hear echo in my head, and soon my body would follow.

Lesson #11:
What A Difference A Year Makes—Keep The Faith.

When the mammogram was over, I was able to go home with peace of mind for another year. I thanked God, once again. Feeling very grateful, the drive home was quick as I anticipated life with my children on a summer day. With the mammogram behind me, I could now focus on a much-needed vacation that Rich and I had planned. It would be our first one alone in quite some time.

With a straw hat and sunscreen in hand, we left one week later for a four-day trip to Cabo San Lucas. It was our present to each other after a long year of self-discovery, pain, discomfort, joy, and the most humbling experience I've ever known.

Our trip through Dallas to San Jose del Cabo was perfect. The ride to our resort was quaint as we shared a taxi with some other newly arriving guests. As we approached the resort, I saw nothing but white. Upon strolling into the lobby, it was clear that we had entered paradise. This spectacular open lobby consisted of two beautiful walls that created the backdrop for two mahogany desks, a magnificent chandelier, a telescope, and a thatch roof. From the lobby, we were able to see the pool and the Sea of Cortez. The soft breeze blowing around us was refreshing. This get-away in paradise was just what the doctor had ordered…the doctor, of course, was me.

We were escorted to our suite, and moments later, found ourselves giddy like two school children ready to begin an exciting new adventure. Peeking through the balcony window just outside our suite, was a white L-shaped couch with powder blue pillows overlooking the sea. In front of the couch was a coffee table that consisted of hand-painted ceramic tiles. Two white wicker chairs, a large fern, and a Jacuzzi with two sconces illuminated by a gas flame, completed the arrangement. A wrought iron spiral staircase wound its way up to a second floor balcony where two lounge chairs with white terrycloth cushions greeted us. The balcony was complemented by a large green cactus and aloe plants that were planted in large orange terracotta pots. I wanted to just sit and take it all in. Like love at first sight, I felt my heartstrings tug. The fishy sea air filled my nostrils, the fading hot sun kissed my skin, and the ocean breeze wrapped its warm arms around me.

I am still amazed, I thought, like a child seeing the ocean for the first time, at how beautiful the waves are splashing up on the shoreline; I am still amazed at how many different colors of blue there are in one ocean; and, I am still amazed at how calming the sound of the ocean breeze is. A sound that some people have captured on tape so that they can fall asleep anywhere listening to the gentle pounding of the foam as it lies down on the sand. "Good night," it says. "Sleep tight, dream well, and I will be here in the morning to greet you when you wake, ready to start another day of life's journey."

As I slowly opened my eyes the next morning, there was a quiet sense of peacefulness that enveloped my mind, body, and soul. Coming out of my slumber, I quietly stepped outside onto the balcony as if early morning was some kind of secret and I was the first one to witness the new day's sun. This morning was my secret, my solitude. The sun glistened like sparkles of glitter on the ocean as the waves had not yet receded from the shoreline. Realizing that this might be the only time all day that I may be completely alone, I savored the moment and held it still in my heart as if it were a buried treasure. I felt an overwhelming rush of coming home, yet, I could not have been farther away. Once again, I thanked God.

Rich and I slowly moved around the resort cherishing the free time we had been given. Feeling completely vulnerable, and yet, empowered at the same time, I vowed to use my experience as a means to embrace and help others. The backdrop of the Sea of Cortez became my canvas, and my battle with breast cancer became my tools to paint a picture of hope and love. The hope for a brighter tomorrow and the love you give to yourself.

Once we had enveloped all there was to take in focusing on relaxing, recharging, rebuilding, re-discovering, re-cooperating, and rejuvenating, it was time to go home. Thanking God for creating such a paradise, we agreed to return again.

****

My prayer for you: Dear God, please grant the reader the awareness to take this unfortunate situation and turn it around to become a blessing in disguise. Help her to remain open to You and all the angels on this Earth she will meet who offer her compassion. May Your goodness be a sense of comfort, the blanket of hope that keeps her close to You. May she never lose faith and have the confidence to go out and offer compassion to others, thereby making this world a better place one person at a time. Amen.

CHAPTER TWELVE

The Journey Continues

Fast forward – May 2011. Life had started to pick up speed as I began taking on too many commitments. Unfortunately, this meant less time spent with God. One day in my haste and stupidity, I suffered an injury to my right elbow which resulted in nerve damage, bicep overuse and tendonitis. Unable to carry on my activities of daily living, let alone teach classes, I was devastated. My world came to a screeching halt. Once again, I brought God back into my life front and center. By June of 2011, I had cleared my calendar, turned my classes over to other instructors and with God's help, focused on healing.

I set up appointments to meet with different doctors. I began acupuncture, ultrasound massage, and finally physical therapy to try to get my arm to heal. X-rays looked good and so did the MRI. The best advice I was given was to take over-the-counter pain medication and to rest it. ARE YOU KIDDING ME? This is my right arm we're talking about. How can I rest it? By turning my eyes to The Lord, I found comfort in knowing that God was with me in my time of need. Deciding to use this opportunity as down time I could once again, focus on prayer, and perhaps, a new direction for my life. I didn't go looking for some "down time", so instead, I chose this time to develop a closer relationship with Jesus and The Blessed Mary. With my mind made up to think positively, I decided to enjoy the summer and my time at home with my children.

By the time summer was over, I had learned to enjoy my new-found freedom once again! I made it a point to start the day with giving thanks and praise to God. Daily prayer took the place of my exercise classes and I realized just how much I had missed spending time in silent prayer.

With my resistance down, pneumonia found a way to creep itself into my life in early December. Forced to lay in bed to get rest, I prayed harder than I had ever prayed before, not thinking that was even possible. By the middle of the second week of being sick in bed, I told my husband, Rich, that if I wasn't better by the next morning, I was going to the hospital. Once again, I turned my heart over to The Lord praying that God would allow me to get better soon.

"Three times I begged the Lord about this, that it might leave me," but He said to me, "My grace is sufficient for you, for power is made perfect in weakness. I will rather boast most gladly of my weaknesses, in order that the power of Christ may dwell in me. Therefore, I am content with weaknesses, insults, hardships, persecutions, and constraints, for the sake of Christ; for when I am weak, then I am strong."—II Corinthians 12:8-10 [12]

As it has been said, The Lord works in mysterious ways! By having complete bed rest for two weeks, guess what? My arm had completely healed…or so I thought. Just before Christmas I was back on my feet and feeling great. I contacted a few clubs that I had worked for and advised them that I would be back teaching after the first of the year.

When January came, I found myself working at the park district and subbing at one the clubs I used to work for. Just two weeks into teaching, I made a terrible mistake. In my zealousness, I lifted a weight that was too heavy and re-injured my arm. WHAT WAS I THINKING? Where was my patience? Once again, I had to back off teaching. This time I was angry. It's easy to pray to God when we're suffering and that's what I realized. When I returned to work, I wasn't putting God first anymore. My focus shifted back to my fitness goals and my daily activities. Realizing just how important daily prayer is, I returned my focus back on Him.

Lesson #12: Keep Your Eyes Fixed On The Lord

God loves us and wants us to turn to Him always. He doesn't want us to forget Him or push Him aside or only call on Him when we need something or when it's convenient. He wants to have a daily relationship with us, and not just when we're hurting.

Philippians 4:6-7 "Don't worry about anything, but in all your prayers ask God for what you need, always asking him with a thankful heart. And God's peace, which is far beyond human understanding, will keep your hearts and minds safe in union with Christ Jesus." [13]

I was learning the hard way to be patient and to keep my trust in God. Like Jonah, I had been hiding from God.

The Book of Jonah: 1:3. "But Jonah made ready to flee to Tarshish away from the Lord." [14]

It's not that Jonah was afraid of The Lord, he worshiped Him and he was God's servant.

"I worship the Lord, the God of heaven, who made the sea and the dry land." Jonah: 1:9 [15]

However, God had plans for Jonah and Jonah resisted. He tried running away from God.

The point I'm trying to make is that when we learn to trust God and put our lives in His hands, the burdens our society places on our shoulders will be lifted. There is a wooden sign in my house that reads, "Relax, God Is In Control." Remember, no matter what, we can't hide from God.

★★★★★★★★★★★★★★★

My prayer for you: Dear God, please help this beautiful reader during her trials and tribulations. Let her breathe deeply and relax and she learns to relinquish control over to you. Help her to be patient with herself and with those around her. May her heart stir and be filled with the Holy Spirit as abundant blessings are placed in her life. I ask this through Christ, Our Lord. Amen.

CHAPTER THIRTEEN

Digging Deeper Into My Faith

With my arm now in need of being "fixed", I turned to physical therapy. Once again, I had to step away from teaching classes. Since I was no longer working, I had plenty of time for prayer. I decided to step my prayer time up a notch and began attending the 9:00 a.m. mass a few times during the week. I was trying real hard to listen for God's voice. On the days I was not at mass, I turned on the small radio in my kitchen where it was programmed to an AM radio station that was primarily Christian talk. I listened to several preachers read from the Bible and give their sermons filled with Bible stories. The more I heard, the more I wanted to know. Hungry for scripture, I invited a few of my favorite radio preachers into my email account by becoming a subscriber. This way, I would also receive daily messages highlighting scripture.

One afternoon during my daily prayer with God, I was gazing out my bedroom window. I felt a strong tug in my heart to become involved in the 9:00 a.m. mass at my church. Since I was already a lector for occasional Sunday masses, I felt it a natural calling to read from the ambo another day during the week. God is so good, I thought. I knew I had time to read any day during the week since I was no longer working.

The following day, I approached a few of the women who attend mass every day and are also the weekly lectors. Expressing my interest, I offered my services. Although I had any day during the week open, that was not God's plan. You see, the only day that there was a need for another 9:00

a.m. reader was on Saturday. The ladies were so happy that someone had volunteered to help them and Saturday was where they needed help. "Could you do that, they asked?" Sure, I said. Great! It was all set. In two weeks I'd begin reading on Saturdays. I walked out of the church that day, looked up at the sky and said, "Well, God, that's not what I had in mind but I guess that's where you need me right now!"

****

One day, my arm was exceptionally painful and I began to lose hope. Angry that it might never heal, I lashed out at God. I was speaking aloud in an angry tone, I was crying, and I threw myself on my bed like a child throwing a temper-tantrum. Did God not hear my pleas to heal my arm? Did God not know that I was going to church more and that I wanted to follow Jesus? If so, why was I still suffering? To calm myself down, I picked up one of the prayer pamphlets next to my bed and I began to read. Next, I picked up my rosary and began to pray. Through my prayer, my body had finally responded by acquiring a sense of calm and peace. No longer was I crying. I felt like the Apostle, Paul, when he said,

"Three times I asked the Lord to remove the thorn that it might depart from me. And he said to me, my grace is sufficient for you; for my strength is made perfect in weakness." II Corinthians 12:8-9 [16].

Emotionally, I picked myself up and realized that I was trying to call the shots. I was trying to control when I should be healed and I was angry that God wasn't answering my prayer for a quick recovery when I wanted it healed. Instead, I decided to pray that God would give me the grace to accept my slow recovery with patience. Once again, I gave up my will to God's will and I surrendered. Embarrassed by my lack of trust and the willfulness to try and control my destiny, I was humbled. No one knew. It was just between God and me.

Peeling myself from my bed, I went to take a hot shower. The moisture in the shower was slowly beginning to steam up the glass shower door and I noticed what appeared to be a picture on the lower portion of the shower door. It looked like a heart that was bleeding due to the line that was running down from the lowest point of it. As the steam began to rise up, another image presented itself. Visible about a foot higher than the bleeding heart, was a small diagonal cross. Ok, I thought, these are signs. God knows my heart is aching (the bleeding heart) and by showing me a cross, He wants me to know that He hears me and is with me. The symbol of the cross is the hope of Jesus. Although I began to feel better, I also felt a bit guilty. I thought about the Apostle Simon Peter during the storm when Jesus was walking on the water.

Simon Peter asked Jesus, "Lord if it is really you order me to come out on the water to meet you." Jesus said, "Come." So Peter left the boat and began walking on the water. When Peter noticed the strong wind, he was afraid and started to sink down in the water. He called out to Jesus to save him. Jesus extended a hand and said, "Oh you of little faith, why did you doubt? Matthew 14:22-31[17]

Amazingly, one more "sign" came into focus. This time, God reminded me to believe in Him with the image of a leaf from my favorite tree, the Beech. As you read in an earlier chapter of this book, a Beech leaf somehow had fallen into the back of my shirt one day. I never felt it and didn't know it was there until bedtime. When my young daughters and I were trying to figure out the significance of all the "gifts" God had given me, we discovered that His message was for us to Bee – Leaf, to BELIEVE in Him.

Overwhelmed by these new "gifts" on my shower door, I began to cry. This time they were happy tears and once again, I felt so blessed. From that moment on, I realized that God's plan will be revealed in His time, not mine. Boy, how quickly I had forgotten that. God has a plan for you too. If we start the day with God on our minds and His love in our hearts, then we can look at the world through God's eyes with the grace He will bestow upon us through the Holy Spirit.

The next day, the heart was gone, but the cross and leaf were still there. Realizing that my own heart no longer felt broken, I was not surprised by its absence on my shower door. I was happy to see that the cross and the leaf were still there, though. As the week progressed, eventually both had disappeared.

****

One day I received an invitation to have lunch with one of my best friends from high school. In our forty+ years of knowing each other, we never really talked about our faith. However, lately, we had been getting together quite a bit for lunch and it only seemed fitting to share my eagerness for the Gospel with her and my excitement about this book. I felt safe with her because she understood me. Over the years, we had confided in each other about several things that had happened in our lives. Things we wouldn't want to discuss with other people for fear we'd be judged. God is amazing! He has a mighty plan! He brings people together when they need it most. Sometimes months before we realize it. She completely understood my excitement with developing a relationship with God and knowing Jesus because, she too, was recently experiencing the same thing. Wow! What a blessing to discover that our relationship had just reached new heights. Beaming, we both sat across the table from one another not saying a word for a few seconds as we realized the direction of where our relationship was heading. We were like two school girls giddy with excitement because we had discovered our true acceptance of one other on a spiritual level. We continued meeting for lunch as often as we could and, at some point, our conversation would always drift toward God.

During one particular lunch in mid-February of 2012, she looked at me a little strange. Wait a minute, I thought. I know that look. The first thing I thought was that I had said something to offend her. Quickly I asked her what was wrong. She turned her head slightly and asked, "Would you ever consider going to a women's weekend retreat." "Yes, I said. Actually I've thought about it several times, why?" "There's a women's retreat in two weeks at my parish and I was invited to go, but I don't want to go by myself. I would love it if you would go with me," she said. I was thrilled! In checking my calendar, it turned out that the weekend was open and so I marked it down. It didn't matter to me that I knew nothing about this women's retreat because I trusted God and I heard his call with my heart. It felt right!

Lesson #13:
There's Always Opportunities To Dig Deeper Into Your Faith

When you make God a priority in your life and when you trust that He knows what's better for you, more than you do, you won't be disappointed. God works in mysterious ways and sometimes, in fact most of the time, it's not what you expect. Seriously, when was the last time you prayed to God and turned the control over to Him? For most people, the answer is never. I'm glad that I did.

****

My prayer for you: Father in heaven help this beautiful woman find peace in her day. Fill her heart up with your love and goodness. Help her to find time each day to spend it with You. Please let her be open to Your calling and help her to hear it so that she can develop a relationship with You. Amen.

CHAPTER FOURTEEN

An Answered Prayer

Happy with a new spiritual direction and the women's weekend, I felt focused once again. Not on me physically, but on God and the direction He was taking me. April was upon us and so was the Confirmation of the large group of freshman high school students my husband, Rich, and I were assisting as Confirmation Leaders. We had one speaker to listen to at church, and a week later, one home meeting left to go before the big day. The topic I chose for our last meeting was going to be about Our Blessed Virgin Mary and how to pray the Rosary which Rich and I felt was very important. Armed with a beautiful movie about St. Lucia and a Rosary Prayer Pamphlet, I felt that we had good material to put forth an effective meeting. The question was how to introduce this type of prayer to the teens without turning them off. Prayer after prayer, I asked God to help us with this. It was so important to us that the teens accept praying the Rosary. At our first meeting, we focused on praying the Lord's Prayer and I can't say that it went over as well as I had hoped. Again, we felt it was important that they knew just what it was that they were saying and not just reciting a bunch of words. In my heart, answering the call to be Confirmation Leaders meant teaching the children how to pray. At some point in their lives, they would feel the need to pray. Rich and I wanted them to feel comfortable with prayer and to depend on prayer for anything and everything…w*orry about nothing, prayer about everything.*

Philippians 4:6-7 "Have no anxiety at all, but in everything, by prayer and petition, with thanksgiving, make your requests known to God. Then the peace of God that surpasses all understanding will guard your hearts and minds in Christ Jesus." [18]

The speaker for our last meeting was a gentleman who we had heard a few months earlier so I couldn't imagine that his topic would be new. As Rich and I sat there in church, the first words out of the speaker's mouth just about knocked me off the pew. He said he was now "into Mary". Sitting up straight and tall, he definitely had my attention. He repeated himself and said that he now prays the Rosary. He raised his hands and low and behold he was holding several handmade Rosaries for all the teens. As Rich and I and the other Confirmation Leaders helped pass out the Rosaries and some pamphlets that he had provided, my eyes were filling up with tears. Wow! What a surprise. Never in a million years would I have imagined just how God would answer my prayer. This gentleman, whom the kids were drawn to, was the perfect introduction to what I wanted to do the following week. Thank you God, you are truly amazing!

Lesson #14: God Hears Our Prayers

The Bible mentions several times that we are to be courageous, strong and not to be afraid. All too often we try and carry the weight of the world on our shoulders. We worry about everything, most of which are things that are not in our control. Learning to lean on God for help and truly believing that He hears our prayers, really does make a big difference in how you perceive the outcome of a situation.

I have received so many blessings in disguise as a result of my diagnosis of breast cancer. For joy and sorrow are twin sisters, you can't experience one without the other. Don't dwell on your sorrows, focus on the joys. The emotions of cancer roll their way through your body like waves of soft agony crashing up on the shoreline. But at the end of the day just as the sun sets above the horizon, its brilliance offers us a tranquil sense of strength, peace and hope for a better tomorrow. Remember, every day is a new day and another second chance at life. In the beautiful words of an unknown author, "When you come to the edge of all the light you know and are about to step off into the darkness of the unknown, FAITH is knowing that one of two things will happen—there will be something solid on which to stand, or you will be given wings to fly"…with that I wish you God's speed.

****

My prayer for you: Dear God, help us to find comfort in life's sorrows and struggles that we don't understand by wrapping us in a blanket of hope. Teach us to trust You, and like the mustard seed, let our faith grow strong.

Questions To Think About

Lesson #15: Don't Be Afraid to Ask Questions, Even If It's The Same Question Twice.

The following questions may help you in making decisions about your choice of doctors, cancer treatment, and hospitals:

1. What is the doctor's bedside manner like?
2. How much confidence do you have in this doctor?
3. What is your impression of how the doctor's office is run?
4. Is the staff helpful and do they seem interested in you?
5. Do you need to be at a teaching hospital, an established well-known hospital, or a community hospital to feel comfortable?
6. Do you need to be close to home in case you have to drive yourself for treatments, if necessary?
7. Will family and friends be able to help out if you choose a hospital far away from your home?
8. Do you have references from the doctor's office?
9. Does the doctor see patients on a daily basis whereby he/she stays connected to the human side of surgery?
10. Have you asked questions about the different types of treatment?
11. Do you know what your options are?
12. How is the doctor's attention toward detail? Is that important to you?

13. Is the type of cancer treatment that your doctor is recommending covered by your insurance?
14. How long has the doctor been a surgeon?
15. How comfortable are you with that fact?
16. Is your doctor and hospital of choice part of your insurance network?
17. What questions do you have that are not listed here?

My prayer for you: Dear God, please give the reader the wisdom to approach these decisions prayerfully and with much thought to detail. May the woman preparing for this journey find comfort in all those who will be a part of this journey with her. I pray that she remain focused on healing and making You, oh Lord, a very important part of her life now and always. Amen.

CHAPTER SIXTEEN

Exercises: Post Cancer Treatment

Lesson #16:
Strength Training, Flexibility, and Cardiovascular Exercise Play An Important Role In Maintaining Good Health

Important: First, consult with your doctor before you begin any exercise program. You should not perform these exercises if you are pregnant, have not been cleared by your doctor to engage in a strength training exercise program, or if you do not have your complete range of motion in your upper body. Chapter 4 of this book addresses regaining your range of motion. Also, do not exercise if you have any swelling in the affected area as with having lymphedema. *Again, never begin an exercise program if you do not have full range of motion of your limbs.* It is imperative that you are able to lift your arm(s) up to its fully extended position or very close to it (90%), thus having flexibility, before you begin to strengthen it. Please ask your doctor for a hand-out of range of motion (ROM) exercises or perform the ROM exercises that I have listed in Chapter 4. ROM is imperative before beginning any strength training program.

Also, if you have had a TRAM flap, LAT flap or any type of reconstructive breast surgery, please get clearance from your doctor before beginning any exercise program. You need to know what your contraindications are. It's always a good idea to work with a personal trainer, especially if you've had reconstructive surgery. You can find one by logging on to the Cancer Exercise Specialist website at www.thecancerspecialist.com. If you are not able to find a Cancer Exercise Specialist in your area, then log on to the American Council on Exercise website at www.acefitness.com. It's imperative that you work with someone from an accredited institution like The Cancer Exercise Specialist Institute or The American Council on Exercise, to name a few, and ask for references. If you belong to a gym or club, make sure you discuss your situation with the fitness director so that she/he can match you up with the right personal fitness trainer to meet your needs. Thank you!

When you are cleared by your doctor, then you're ready to begin. I recommend starting with light hand weights (1 or 2 lbs.) You should be able to complete 8 to 10 repetitions of each exercise without feeling pain. *If at any time you feel pain or experience any swelling, please stop the exercise and consult with your doctor.* If 2 lb. hand weights feel too light, then increase the weight in small increments. In this case try 3 lb. weights. You should never jump up in weights too quickly because if you do experience swelling, it would be hard to determine which poundage of weight was too much for your body to handle. If it's too hard to perform 8 to 10 repetitions, then jump back down in weight to the next lightest one.

Ideally, you should be able to build upon your strength so that you can perform at least 12 to 15 repetitions with the last two repetitions being somewhat of a challenge, but not impossible, *while maintaining proper form*. Once you can perform 1 set of 12 – 15 repetitions of a certain weight (example 3 lbs.), then you can build upon that and perform a 2nd set of that weight (3 lbs.) however, you need to drop your repetitions back down to 8 to 10. Slowly increase the 2nd set of repetitions to 12 – 15 before moving on to the next heavier weight (example 4 lbs.) This should be a slow progression taking you about 8 – 12 weeks @ twice per week with 1 to 2 days of rest in between strength training sessions. You want to gradually build on your weight strength over a period of at least 8 weeks before you move up to the next weight. Slow progression is what you need to focus on so that you make progress in the right direction. *As a breast cancer survivor, you need to be concerned with avoiding lymphedema.* It's more important to use less weight and more repetitions than it is to focus on lifting as much heavy weight as possible. There really shouldn't be any need to lift anything heavier than 5 to 8 lb. weights. I only lift 3 – 5 lb. weights myself. Some days I only perform 1 set. Some weeks I only lift weights once that week. My point is, where lifting weights is important to maintaining muscle mass, off-setting osteoporosis, and keeping your metabolism up and running thereby keeping your body weight down, don't stress over it. It's important to focus on your cardio exercise program and to maintain flexibility. Flexibility is key!

Please note: Strength training is not meant as a substitution for cardio fitness exercises such as walking, running, swimming, sports games, and/or dancing. Strength training exercises, just like flexibility exercises, are to be performed in addition to cardiovascular exercises.

Cardiovascular exercise on the other hand, can be performed every day. As a personal trainer, I advise my clients to aim for four to five days a week of cardio exercise for at least thirty to forty-five minutes per session. Most people can fit in three days of cardio exercise into their schedules per week but four or five would be most beneficial. Three to four days a week is a good starting point, however, eventually (within six to eight weeks) work your way up to four or five days of cardio. Intensity will not be discussed in this book as that is based upon the individual's performance ability. Please give yourself at least one day of rest of not exercising at all. I prefer Sundays!

Important: <u>Do Not</u> hold your breath while performing these exercises. Remember to breathe! Exhale on exertion—usually the first movement, the push or the pull. Inhale on the opposite move.

To help get you started, listed below are some examples of basic exercises that work the major muscles of your body. For additional help, there are several books on the market that can help you achieve your goals. Make sure you begin with at least a 5 to 10 minute warm up. Also, *it's important to help reduce the risk of lymphedema by performing deep breathing exercises and the lymph drainage exercises* before beginning your strength training session. For your convenience, I have included the lymph drainage exercises for the upper body in this chapter. Always gently stretch your muscles safely whenever you complete a strength training workout. I have included basic stretches at the end of this chapter. However, you may want to check your local library or favorite book store for more examples of stretches.

Lymph Drainage Exercises for the Upper Body:

Warm Up For The Strength Training Session

Slowly warm the body up first. To do this, I recommend marching in place for about 3 to 5 minutes. Eventually add slow arm circles…5 repetitions moving the arms forward, then 5 moving the arms backwards while maintaining your march. Next, take that march to a little jog in place for a few minutes. You can then add some kicks, hamstring curls, jumping jacks, etc., anything that will get your heart rate up a bit and increase your respiration. Overall, you should have warmed-up for about 5 to 10 minutes.

Once you are warmed-up and feel good, then continue with deep abdominal breathing. Sit down in a comfortable chair sitting up straight with your feet flat on the floor. Place your hands either behind your head or across your shoulders. Take a deep breath in through your nose and slowly blow out through your mouth with pierced lips as if you were going to blow out candles. As you blow out, pull in your abdominal muscles. You should feel your low back come up against the back of the chair as you blow out and pull your abdominal muscles in. Now breathe in and straighten back up. Repeat this about 10 times.

Next, lay down on a mat on your back with your knees bent and your feet flat on the mat to begin pelvic and basic modified crunches.

Pelvic Tilts

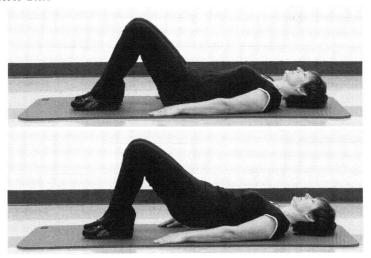

Begin pelvic tilts by laying on a mat on your back with your knees bent, your feet flat on the floor, and your low back snug into the mat. Your head is down on the mat. Keep your chin up and your hands should be down by your sides. Now, slowly lift your hips and butt off the floor while keeping your head and shoulder blades on the mat. Your low back will lift slightly off the mat. Squeeze your glutes (butt) and pause at the highest point of your lift for a few seconds. Then slowly bring your hips/butt back down to the mat and place the low back into the mat by pulling your abdominal muscles in. Perform these pelvic tilts/lifts about 8 – 10 times.

Basic Modified Crunches

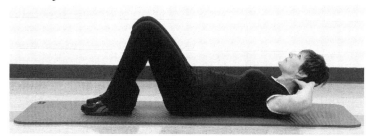

Continue lying on your back on the mat with your head down, feet flat, knees bent, and low back pulled into the mat by pulling your abdominal muscles in. Place your hands behind your head or across your chest if it is not comfortable for you to place your hands behind your head just yet. Slowly lift your head, neck and shoulders (if possible) off the mat as you look straight up toward the ceiling counting to four as you lift. Hold that position for one second before slowly lowering back down to the mat. Maintain your gaze up toward the ceiling throughout the movement. Don't pull on your neck to lift up. Use your abs to do the lifting, even if it feels like you are not lifting very high at all. Keep your low back on the mat. Don't arch your back and don't forget to breathe out as you rise up. Continue the basic modified crunches for at least 8 – 10 repetitions.

By performing pelvic tilts and basic crunches, this will give the lymphatic system from the upper extremities a place to drain in to, thus decreasing the likelihood of lymphedema in the upper extremities. If you had a sentinel node biopsy, or if you have had any lymph nodes removed, you are at risk for lymphedema.

Neck Stretches

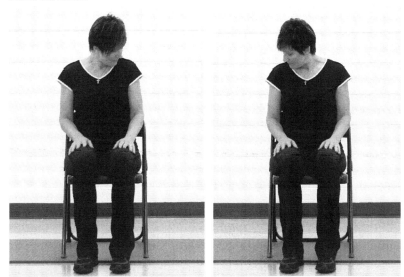

Sit on your mat or a comfortable chair. Roll your shoulders up, back and down to stretch them away from your ears. Next, gently turn your head to the right, back to center, then to the left and back to center (starting position). Exhale while moving your head to the right and left, inhale as you bring your head back to center. Continue the stretches by turning your head to the right and bring your chin down toward your right shoulder. Hold that stretch for 5 seconds before returning to the starting position with your head in the center. Slowly turn your head to the left and lower your chin toward your left shoulder. Hold for 5 seconds before returning your head to the starting position.

Shoulder Shrugs

Inhale while lifting your shoulders toward your ears, exhale and bring your shoulders back down. Repeat about 6 times.

Isometric Shoulder Blade Squeeze

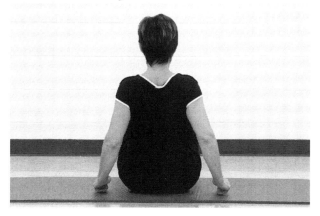

Exhale and slowly pull your shoulder blades down and squeeze them together. Hold that position for a few seconds then release the squeeze. Repeat about 8 times.

Isometric Chest Presses (prayer presses)

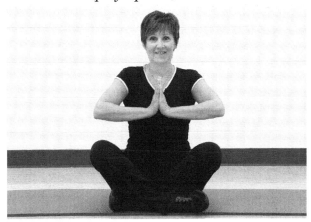

Place the palms of your hands together in front of your chest. Your elbows should be up with your forearms parallel to the floor (basically in a prayer position). Exhale and push the palms of your hands firmly together, hold for a few seconds, and then inhale as you release the tension in your hands. Repeat this 8 times.

Wrist Flexion

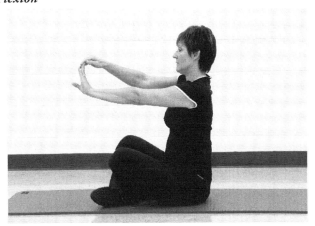

Bring your left arm straight out in front of you at shoulder height and position your hand as if you were telling someone to stop. With your right hand, grab your left fingers and, with gentle tension, slowly bend your wrist back a bit toward your forearm. This will be a very slight movement. Hold that position for 5 seconds then release. Repeat about 8 times with the left arm before switching arms.

Wrist Extension

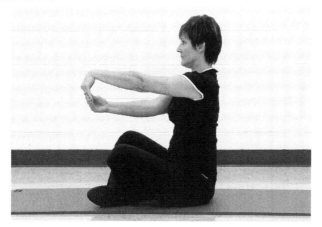

Bring your left arm straight out in front of you at shoulder height and position your hand with your fingers down. With your right hand, grab your left fingers and slowly bend your wrist down (opposite of wrist flexion) as if you were going to have someone kiss the top of your hand... just like in the old days!! This will be a very slight movement. Hold that position for 5 seconds then release. Repeat about 8 times with the left arm before switching arms.

Finger Stretches

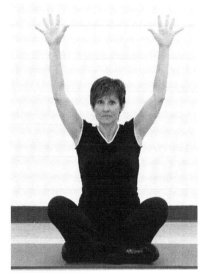 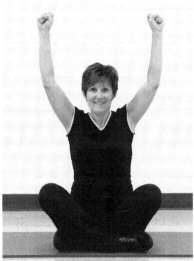

Lift your arms up overhead as high as you comfortably can. Open your hands wide by spreading your fingers apart. Then, close your hands into a fist. Repeat opening and closing your hands slowly about 8 times then lower your arms back down.

Strength Training Exercises:

Legs

Squats: Works your gluteals, hamstrings, and quadriceps, inner thighs and hip flexors muscles.

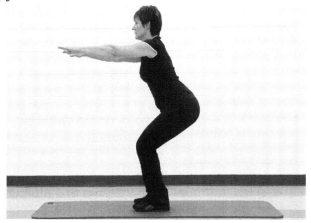

Stand with your legs hips-width apart and your feet facing forward. Slowly bend your knees as you move your butt back as if you were going to sit in a chair, but do not place all your weight in your butt as this may cause you to fall back. Instead, keep your weight shifted forward. Make sure you can see your toes.

You may place your hands on your thighs, or extend them out in front of you to help maintain your balance.

Keep your chest lifted.

Do not squat too low. Position your body so that your butt does not drop lower than your knees.

Pushing through your heels, slowly rise back up to a standing position.

Perform this exercise 10 to 12 times. Pause at the top of the exercise (complete standing position) for a couple of seconds before you repeat the exercise.

Standing Calf Raises: Works your calves – soleus and gastrocnemius muscles.

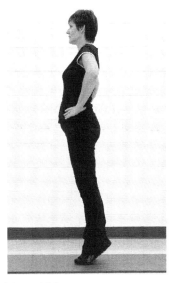

Stand with your legs hips-width apart.

Slowly lift your body upward by lifting your heels off the floor as you rise up on the balls of your feet and toes.

Hold that position for a couple of seconds, then slowly lower back down onto your heels and back to the starting position with your feet flat.

Repeat this exercise 10 to 12 times.

Back

One-Arm Bent Over Rows: Works your trapezius, posterior deltoids, latissimus dorsi, and rhomboids muscles.

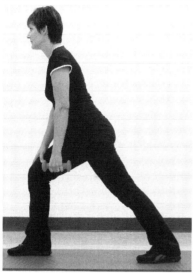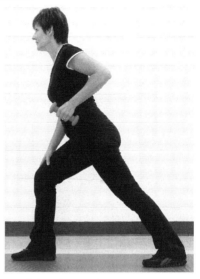

Stand with your feet hips-width apart and feet facing forward.

Place the right leg about two feet in front of the left and hips-width apart. Your feet should look as though they are straddled on railroad tracks.

Lean your bodyweight forward so that the right leg's knee is bent. The back leg (left leg) should be straight, however, keeping the knee slightly bent and the back foot flat.

Place your right on your right thigh just above the knee.

Hold a 3 to 5 lb. hand weight in the palm of your left hand. Grip the weight so that it does not fall out of your hand.

Let the left arm hang down without dropping the shoulder. Keep your shoulders parallel to the floor and your neck in line with your spine.

Slowly lift the left arm up by bending your elbow up toward the ceiling, keeping the elbow close to your body as you bring it up. You should feel a slight retraction of your left shoulder blade.

Keep your back straight, abdominals pulled in, and your neck in line with your spine.

Count for about four seconds as you lift your elbow up, pause at the top of the movement for about one second and slowly lower your hand to the starting position.

Count about four seconds down as you resist gravity.

Perform this exercise about 10 to 12 times.

You need to choose a weight that will allow you to perform the exercise at least ten times, with the last two repetitions becoming a bit challenging, but not impossible, and with perfect form.

Once you have completed 10 to 12 repetitions then switch sides.

Bring your left leg forward and your right leg in back.

Switch arms and place the weight in your right hand.

Continue with lifting the right arm the same way you lifted the left.

Complete this exercise 10 to 12 repetitions then move on to the next exercise.

The following Back Extension/Dorsal Raise should only be performed if you have full range of motion of your arms and if you are comfortable laying on your stomach. If not, skip this exercise and perform the following Dead Lift exercise.

Back Extension/Dorsal Raise: *Works the lower back extensors, upper back, abdominal muscles and gluteal muscles.*

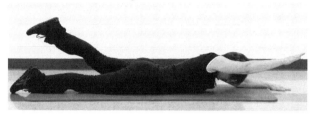

Lie on a mat on your stomach with your head lifted a few inches from the mat.

Extend your arms out in front and over your head as if you are reaching for something on the ground.

Extend your legs straight out behind you and rest your toes on the ground.

Lift your left arm and your right leg off the ground at the same time and hold them in the air for two to three seconds.

Keep both your leg and arm straight.

Lower your left arm and right leg, then switch sides and hold the right arm and left leg up for about two to three seconds.

Continue to alternate lifting your opposite arm and leg for about 10 to 12 repetitions.

Make sure you keep your neck in line with your spine.

Dead Lift: *Works the lower back, gluteal muscles and hamstrings:*

Stand with your feet hips-width apart and holding one weight in each hand and your palms facing the front of your legs.

Slowly bend at your waist and slide the weights down your legs to your knees. Pause, then slowly stand back up sliding the weights back up your legs. To support your spine, make sure you are pulling your abdominal muscles in as you rise. That is one repetition. Perform this exercise (to the top of the knees and back up) three more times.

Next, slowly bend from your waist and slide the weights down your legs a little farther so that the weights are just below the knees. Pause, then slowly stand back up in the same manner as above. Perform this exercise (just below the knees and back up) three more times.

To add to that, slowly bend from your waist and slide the weights down your legs farther down (3/4 way down your legs, but not to your ankles, and back up). Pause, then slowly stand back up sliding the weights back up the legs and holding your abdominal muscles in. Repeat this exercise three more times.

Finally, slowly bend from your waist and slide the weights down your legs to your ankles. Try and do this without bending your knees, however, only if you can reach your ankles without straining. Pause, then slowly stand back up sliding the weights back up your legs to your full and upright standing position. Perform this exercise (to the ankles and back up) three more times.

Chest

Chest Presses: Works your pectorals and shoulder muscles.

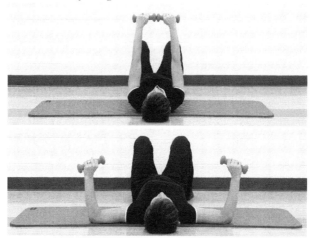

Lay on a mat on your back with your head down and your feet flat on the mat keeping your knees bent.

Hold a 3 to 5 lb. weight in each hand.

Lift the weights straight up in the air with your arms resembling the number 11, in other words, straight up, hands separated and directly over your chest, not over your neck or head. Keep the arms straight with the back of your hand facing you, your palms facing away from you. Don't lock out the elbows, keep them slightly bent.

Slowly bend your elbows, separating your hands, as you bring your arms down toward the mat positioning the top half of your arms (specifically the triceps) on the mat to form a goal post position. Your hands will be off the ground and facing upward (your rings to the ceiling).

Pause for a second then slowly lift your arms straight up and over your chest again bringing the weights close together.

Repeat this exercise for about 10 to 12 repetitions.

Again, make sure you can comfortably perform at least ten repetitions, with the last two becoming a bit challenging, but not impossible.

Keep a pace of about four seconds down, pause for a second or two, and then push the weights back up in about three to four seconds. Do not lock your elbows at the top of the exercise.

Biceps

*Bicep curls: **Works the biceps and forearms.***

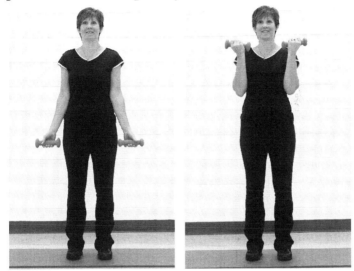

Stand with your feet hips-width apart with your feet forward and knees slightly bent and not locked.

Hold a 3 to 5 lb. weight in each hand.

Place your arms all the way down by your sides with your palms facing out.

Keep your elbows close to your sides and tucked into your hips as you slowly bend the elbows bringing the weights up toward your shoulders.

Your shoulders should not be moving with this exercise. The motion comes from bending the elbows and contracting the biceps.

Count a pace of about four seconds to bring the weights up to your shoulders.

Pause at the top and count about four seconds as you bring the weights all the way down to the starting position.

Perform about 10 to 12 repetitions.

As previously stated, you should be able to perform at least ten repetitions without pain, however, the last two repetitions should seem a bit challenging, but not impossible and with good form.

Triceps

Triceps Extension: Works the triceps muscles.

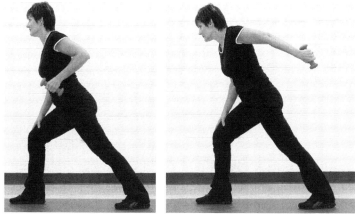

Stand with your feet hips-width apart.

Place the right leg about two feet in front of the left and hips-width apart. Your feet should look as though they are straddled on railroad tracks.

Lean your bodyweight forward so that the right leg's knee is bent. The back leg (left leg) should be straight, however, keeping the knee slightly bent and the back foot flat.

Place your right on your right thigh just above the knee.

Hold a 3 to 5 lb. hand weight in the palm of your left hand. Grip the weight so that it does not fall out of your hand.

Let the left arm hang down without dropping the shoulder. Keep your shoulders parallel to the floor and your neck in line with your spine.

Slowly lift the left arm up by bending your elbow. Keep the elbow close to your body as you continue to lift the elbow up toward the ceiling as high as possible. *This is your starting position.*

Without moving your shoulder, extend your elbow behind you while you bring the weight behind you and straighten out your arm. Your palm is facing your body.

Hold for one second and bring the weight back in toward your body by bending the elbow and moving the weight back toward your ribs and shoulder, without dropping or moving your shoulder.

Repeat this exercise for 10 to 12 repetitions before switching arms.

Shoulders

Front Raises: Works the anterior deltoid.

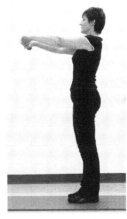

Stand with your feet hips-width apart, facing forward, and your knees slightly bent and not locked.

Hold a 3 to 5 lb. weight in each hand with your palms facing the front of your legs.

Slowly lift your arms straight out in front of you, keeping your elbows straight, but not locked.

Don't lift the weights any higher than your shoulders.

Count four seconds as you lift and four seconds as you lower the weights all the way back down to the starting position.

Repeat this exercise about 10 to 12 times.

Pay close attention to how your shoulders feel at the top of the exercise. If you feel any discomfort or pain, then reduce the amount of weight you are holding. You should be able to perform about ten repetitions without pain or discomfort and with perfect form.

Lateral Raises: Works the medial deltoid.

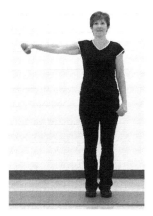

Stand with your feet hips-width apart, facing forward, and with your knees slightly bent and not locked.

Hold a 3 to 5 lb. weight in each hand with your palms facing toward the sides of your legs.

Slowly lift <u>one arm at a time</u> straight out to the side, keeping your elbows straight, but not locked.

Don't lift the weights any higher than your shoulders.

Count four seconds as you lift and about four seconds as you lower the weights all the way back down to the starting position.

Repeat this exercise about 10 to 12 times with one arm before switching arms.

Pay close attention to how your shoulders feel at the top of the exercise. If you feel any discomfort or pain, then reduce the amount of weight you are holding. You should be able to perform about ten repetitions without pain or discomfort, and with perfect form.

Abdominals

Basic Crunches: Works the rectus abdominis muscle.

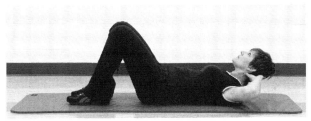

Lay with your back on a mat, head down, feet flat and knees bent.

Place your hands behind your head.

Slowly lift your head, neck and shoulders (if possible) off the mat counting to four as you lift.

Hold your head, neck and shoulders (if possible) off the mat for one second before slowly lowering them back down to the mat.

Maintain your gaze up toward the ceiling throughout the movement.

Don't pull on your neck to lift up. Use your abs to do the lifting, even if it feels like you are not lifting very high at all.

You can place one hand on your abs to feel the muscle engaged.

Keep you low back on the mat. Don't arch your back.

And don't forget to breathe out as you rise up.

Continue lifting your head, neck and shoulders off the mat for at least 15 repetitions.

Reverse Crunch: Works the transverse abdominis and hip flexor muscles.

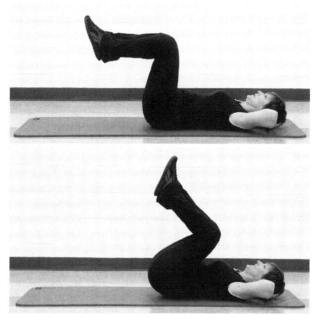

Lay with your back on a mat, head down, feet flat and knees bent.

Place your hands behind your head, or place them down at your sides.

Keep your upper body down on the mat as you lift your feet off the mat, bringing the knees in toward your chest.

Keep your knees bent so that they resemble a 90 degree angle.

Continue to slowly bring your knees in toward your chest as you lift your hips off the floor.

Continue lifting your hips off the mat for 15 repetitions.

Note: If you are having a hard time lifting your hips off the mat, then just bring your knees in toward your chest. You may rock your knees in to your chest, using momentum to lift the hips, but be careful not to strain. Eventually try and eliminate the rocking so that you can use the transverse abdominis (lower abs) muscle to do the lifting. Another option would be to bring your left leg up toward your chest, while the right foot is on the mat, keeping the knee bent. Then bring the right leg up toward your chest and place the left foot on the mat. Keep alternating legs as if you were marching.

Clamshell Crunches: Works the rectus and transverse abdominis muscle, as well as, the hip flexors.

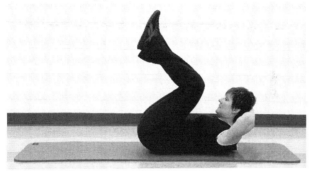

Combine the Basic Crunch with the Reverse Crunch.

Lay on your back on a mat.

Start by keeping your upper body down on the mat, as you lift your feet off the mat, keeping your knees bent so that they resemble a 90 degree angle.

Place your hands behind your head.

While lifting your head, neck and shoulders off the mat, simultaneously lift your hips by drawing your knees in to your chest, bringing your upper and lower body together like a clamshell.

Once you lift your shoulder blades and hips together, hold that position for one second, then slowly return your head down to the mat and bring your hips down at the same time so that the legs remain bent and in the starting position of a 90 degree angle.

Repeat clamshell crunches for 15 repetitions.

Bicycle: Works the rectus and transverse abdominis muscles, as well as, the internal and external obliques.

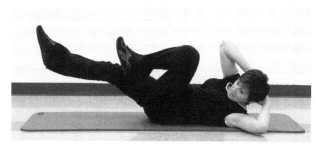

Lay with your back on a mat, head down, knees bent in a 90 degree angle, feet off the floor, and hands behind your head.

Extend your right leg straight out and in front of you. Keep your right leg lifted up slightly higher than your hip (unless you feel discomfort in your low back, then raise your leg up a bit more until you no longer feel discomfort in your low back).

Lift your head, neck, and shoulders off the floor and twist your upper body to bring your right elbow in the direction of the left knee that is pulled in toward your chest (obviously your left foot is off the ground).

Switch by pulling your right leg in toward your chest and extend the left leg straight out while simultaneously twisting the upper body to allow the left elbow to reach toward the right knee.

Continue to twist and hold for one second, keeping your head, neck and shoulders off the mat throughout the exercise. *Repeat alternating knees and elbows for 15 repetitions.

Basic Stretches

Hamstrings/Calves with the addition of the Hips/Glutes Stretch:

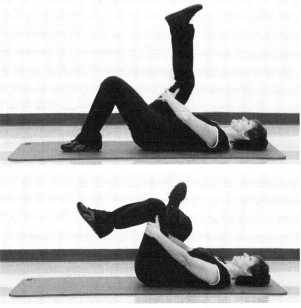

Lay on a mat on the floor, carpet or your bed without pillows (mat/floor preferred) on your back with your feet flat and your knees bent. Keep your head down. Lift your right leg up and hold your leg up with your hands positioned behind the knee. Hold your leg up straight for 30 seconds. Next, while keeping your leg in that position, rotate your ankles about 8 times in each direction. If you can, flex your foot (point the toe down toward your shin bone) and hold the foot in that position for about 15 – 30 seconds. You should feel a stretch in the back of your leg between your heel and back of the knee. Release the foot and keep it neutral (normal position). Next, use your hands to bring your leg in toward your body a little closer without feeling pain. Hold that position for another 30 seconds. *To stretch the hips and glutes*, cross your right leg over your left by placing your right foot on top of the left knee. Slightly press the right leg away from your body. Next, wrap your hands around the left thigh and bring both legs in toward your chest. In doing so, your hips will be lifted off the mat/bed a bit. You should feel a nice stretch in the hips/glutes of the right leg. Hold that stretch for 30 seconds. Uncross the right leg and place it back down keeping the foot flat on the floor and the knee bent. Now lift the left leg and repeat the hamstring/calf stretch, with the addition of the hips/glutes.

Abdominal Stretch:

While laying on a mat, carpet, or your bed without pillows on your back, (mat/floor preferred) place your arms overhead and as far down on the ground as you can. If you need to bend your elbows and bring your hands closer to your head while trying to keep them on the ground, please do, however, your goal should be to get those arms up over your head. Straighten out your legs and reach your arms and legs away from your torso as if you were on a stretching machine. Hold that stretch for 30 seconds.

Supine Floor Stretch/Chest Stretch:

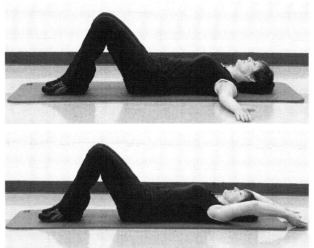

Lay down on your back on either a mat, carpet, or your bed without pillows. Raise your arms up perpendicular to your body and then lay them down over your head. Keeping your arms to the floor or bed, slowly bring your arms away from your head forming a letter T. Hold that stretch for about 30 seconds drawing your shoulder blades together and open/stretch your chest.

Back Stretch:

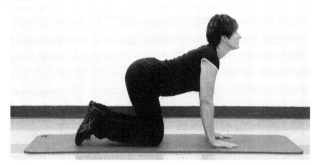

While kneeling on a mat on the floor or carpet, place your hands also on the mat or carpet. Make sure that your hands are placed about two feet in front of your knees so that your hands and elbows are lined up underneath your shoulders and that your knees are lined up underneath your hips. Pushing your hands into the mat or carpet, pull your abs in and up so that your back is rounded. Your head and neck should be in line with your spine in a straight line. Your eyes should be looking down. Now blow out through your mouth and hold that "cat stretch" for about 15 seconds. Then reverse the move by gently breathing in, lift your head up and arch your back by bringing your belly button toward the mat or carpet. Do not bend your elbows. You want to keep the arms taut. Repeat this rounding and arching of the back about 10 times.

Shoulder/Tricep Stretch:

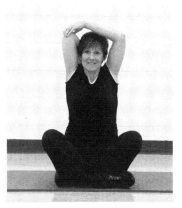

While seated on a mat or carpet with your legs crossed and sitting comfortably, extend your right arm across your body and hold it in place with your left hand. Hold for 15 seconds. Next reach both arms up overhead. Bend the right elbow, dropping your hand and placing your palm on the back of your head. Place the left hand on the right elbow and slowly move the right arm back behind your head as far as you comfortably can without pulling or feeling pain. Your right hand should move slightly down toward your shoulder blade. Hold that pose for 15 seconds then switch arms beginning with placing the left arm across the body for the shoulder.

Overhead Side Bends/Bicep Stretch:

Stand with your feet hips-width apart. Reach your arms up overhead. Clasp your hands together and slowly bend your waist to one side while keeping your hands clasped and arms stretched overhead. Hold that position for 15 to 30 seconds. Stand straight back up while keeping your arms up and back to center over your head (starting position). Next, slowly bend your waist to the other side bringing your arms into a side bend stretch to the other side and hold that position for 15 to 30 seconds. Bring your arms down and next to your sides. Next, and to stretch the biceps, extend the right arm behind you leading with your baby "pinky" finger, turn your head back to follow the right hand. Now turn your arm so that the right thumb is up and continue to bring your arm as far back as possible. Hold for 15 seconds. You should feel a stretch in the shoulder, but primarily the bicep. Repeat the bicep stretch with the left arm.

Quadricep Stretch:

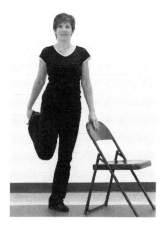

Lastly, the stretch the quadriceps, hold on to the back of a chair. Lift your right foot behind you toward your butt and hold the right foot with your right hand to gently bring the foot up closer to your glutes. Do not lean forward. Stand up straight with your abdominal muscles pulled in. Hold the quad stretch for 30 seconds. Repeat the stretch on the other side bringing your left foot up toward your glutes and holding it with your left hand.

Never hold a stretch beyond what your body is capable of allowing you to do. You should never feel pain. You may, however, feel some tightness and that's ok. Excruciating pain is not acceptable.

Remember to always breathe. Do not hold your breath.

The following sources have been used as a reference to the exercises included in this chapter:
The American Academy of Health & Fitness Training Series[19]
Women's Strength Training Anatomy[20]

****

My prayer for you: Dear God, please give the reader the opportunity to perform these strength exercises to the best of her ability and with proper form. Please help her make strength gains so that she can work toward her goal. Help her come to rely on her newfound strength so that she can become a positive example for the women in her life. Amen.

Bibliography

Bible Source: Saint Joseph Edition of The New American Bible, Catholic Book Publishing Corp., New Jersey

Bible Source: Good News Bible, Good News Translation, American Bible Society, New York, Today's English Version-Second Edition 1992.

Chapter 1
1. 1. Scripture Index: Romans 14:7-12
2. 2. Scripture Index: Hebrews 12:1-3

Chapter 2
3. Scripture Index: John 20:24-29
4. Scripture Index: Matthew 14:27-31
5. Scripture Index: II Corinthians, 12:8-10.

Chapter 4
6. Cancer Exercise Specialist Studyguide/Handbook, 8th Edition. Andrea Leonard, B.A., C.S.C.S., C.P.T., CES along with Dr. Glenn B. Gero – Conquering Cancer with Nutrition and Dr. Joseph Camp – Pilates.

Chapter 5
7. Scripture Index: Matthew 7:7.
8. Scripture Index: Luke 11:9.
9. Scripture Index: Mark 11:24.

Chapter 9
    10. Scripture Index: Matthew 11:28-30
    11. Scripture Index: Hebrews 11:1; 6-7; 11:11

Chapter 12
    12. Scripture Index: II Corinthians 12:8-10
    13. Scripture Index: Philippians 4:6-7
    14. Scripture Index: Jonah 1:3
    15. Scripture Index: Jonah 1:9

Chapter 13
    16. Scripture Index: II Corinthians 12:8-9
    17. Scripture Index: Matthew 14:22-31

Chapter 14
    18. Scripture Index: Philippians 4:6-7

Chapter 16
    19. The American Academy of Health & Fitness Training Series, Tammy J. Petersen, M.S.E., copyright 2008, various tips between pages 163 through 181.
    20. Women's Strength Training Anatomy, Frederic Delavier, (Human Kinetics, Champaign, IL, copyright 2003).

About the Author

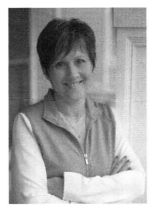

Linda Hillsman is married and has three children. She has been an American Council on Exercise (ACE) Certified Personal Fitness Trainer since 2002, specializing as a Senior Fitness Trainer through The American Academy of Health and Fitness since 2009. Traveling to Miami in 2003, she became licensed as a Zumba Instructor from the creator of Zumba, Beto Perez, bringing Latin-inspired music and fitness moves to the Chicagoland area. Since that time, her fitness accomplishments include: Zumba Toning, Zumba Gold, Aqua Zumba; Les Mills Body Pump; Group Fitness Certification through The Aerobics and Fitness Association of America (AFAA); PILOXING; and her most recent accomplishment was becoming accredited as a Cancer Exercise Specialist.

Linda has been a breast cancer survivor since 2002. After her mastectomy, she was faced with the challenge of regaining range of motion to the affected side of her body. Hard work and determination helped Linda overcome her physical obstacles. She brings this passion for remaining healthy and fit to her personal training clients, as well as, to her class participants. Her love for God and prayers to Him, through Jesus Christ our Lord and the Blessed Virgin Mary, have given her the courage to share her story with other women. A Blanket of Hope Through Faith & Fitness was written to offer support to women suffering from breast cancer and to encourage them to reach out to God. Faith comes from knowing that you are not alone in this fight and that God will always be with you every step of your journey. Comfort comes from feeling the loving arms of Jesus wrapped around you like a blanket of hope.

19021829R00089

Made in the USA
San Bernardino, CA
09 February 2015